Satisfyin

# plant powered athlete

**Written by Zuzana Fajkusova and
photographed by Nikki Lefler**

Founders of Active Vegetarian

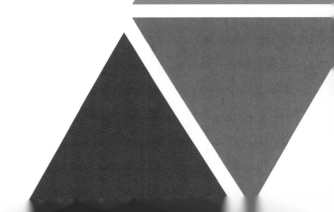

PAGE STREET
PUBLISHING CO.

## PAGE STREET
PUBLISHING CO.

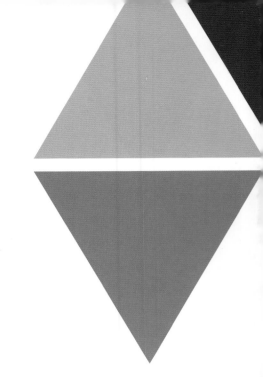

First published in 2020 by
Page Street Publishing Co.
27 Congress Street, Suite 105
Salem, MA 01970
www.pagestreetpublishing.com

Distributed by Macmillan, sales in Canada by The Canadian Manda Group.

24  23  22  21  20    1  2  3  4  5

ISBN-13: 978-1-64567-028-5
ISBN-10: 1-64567-028-7

Library of Congress Control Number: 2019951269

Cover and book design by Molly Gillespie for Page Street Publishing Co.
Photography by Nikki Lefler. Photos on pages 31, 45, 46, 68, 94, 215 & 218 by Jenna Jones

Printed and bound in China

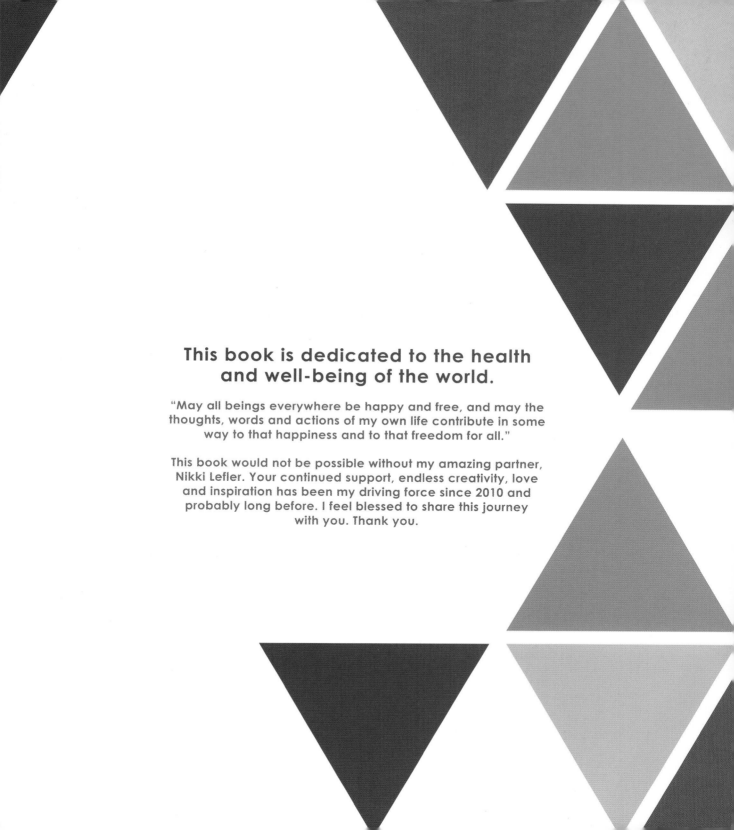

**This book is dedicated to the health and well-being of the world.**

"May all beings everywhere be happy and free, and may the thoughts, words and actions of my own life contribute in some way to that happiness and to that freedom for all."

This book would not be possible without my amazing partner, Nikki Lefler. Your continued support, endless creativity, love and inspiration has been my driving force since 2010 and probably long before. I feel blessed to share this journey with you. Thank you.

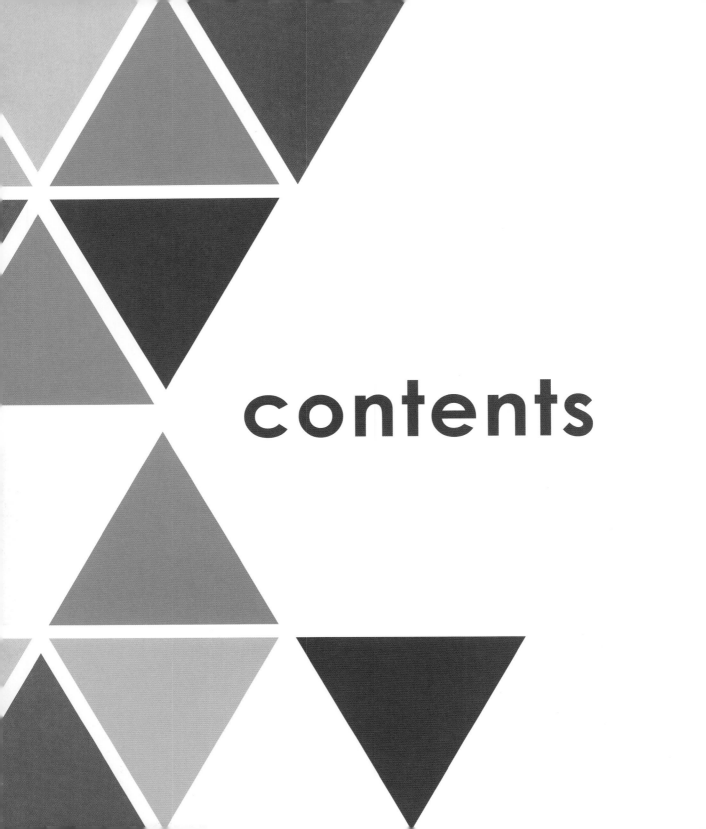

# contents

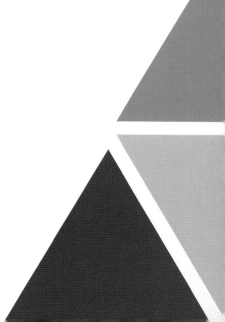

# introduction

All life on earth emanates from the green of the plant.
—Jay Kordich

Today's world of fitness and nutrition can be very confusing and misleading. Authors, companies and products continue to complicate things and promote a shortsighted approach to health. We have been conditioned to go after six-pack abs and overnight miracles without putting in much effort. Many people would do anything to reach their goals, even if it means sacrificing their health and longevity. High-protein, low-carb diets, expensive supplements, products that claim to burn fat while you sleep—sure, some of these could deliver results, but at what cost to your health?

The only way to build a healthy, active, muscular and lean body is through eating and living naturally.

Plant-based diets are becoming popular these days and rightfully so. Elimination of animal protein, refined and chemical-laden foods gives you the potential to shed excess weight, build strength, increase energy and dramatically improve your health and overall well-being. But only if done right! Eating processed food (even if it's labelled "vegan") is not the answer! Vibrant health and peak athletic performance are impossible if you're eating processed food. If you are interested in eating a healthy, sustainable plant-based diet that supports your active lifestyle, this book will help you get there.

Whole, organic plant-based foods have the most amount of nutrition and the least amount of calories. These foods are "living" and come packed with vitamins, minerals, enzymes and antioxidants that are essential for optimal health and peak athletic performance. Living plant foods are also alkaline-forming, which helps reduce inflammation as well as enhancing bone health and immunity, among other amazing benefits.

## Results You Can Expect from the Plant-Powered Diet

- Less digestive stress
- Improved energy levels
- Diminished cravings
- Faster recovery from exercise
- Reduced body fat
- Greater ability to build healthy muscle tissue
- Increased strength and stamina
- More restful sleep and less need for sleep
- Enhanced memory, mental clarity and power of concentration
- Ability to focus more clearly
- Better and younger-looking skin

## The Paradigm Shift

It's common knowledge these days that fast food (e.g., burgers and fries), junk food (e.g., potato chips), processed carbohydrates (e.g., white bread and doughnuts) and sugary drinks (e.g., soda) are not the kinds of food you want to eat for weight loss, health and athletic performance.

However, many people are still unsure of what a healthy diet is supposed to look like. Are carbs good or bad? Do I have to fast for most of the day to lose weight? Should I be putting butter in my coffee? Conflicting messages by companies and self-proclaimed experts (with convincing social media messages and big advertising budgets) are contributing to nutritional confusion that is leading the consumer down a dark rabbit hole.

So many athletes and weekend warriors are making the costly mistake of consuming the wrong kind of food. Instead of supporting their bodies and the work they put in during training, they jeopardize their health and hinder their performance. Personally, I had to learn the truth the hard way. When I began my fitness journey back in 1995, I followed the recommendations from popular books and magazines that emphasized the importance of eating lots of protein, preferably from animal sources. After several months of training hard, drinking protein shakes and eating a "clean" muscle-building diet, I started to experience some unpleasant changes in my health. I stopped menstruating and was dealing with acne and a skin rash that was affecting my self-image. I also felt tired all the time, and it took a tremendous amount of effort to get through my training sessions. Then in 1996, I became a vegetarian after learning about the inhumane practices that are often involved in raising animals for food. I began with eliminating meat from my diet and replaced it with eggs, dairy, tofu and vegan alternatives. Shortly after that, I noticed a slight improvement in my health.

My energy levels improved and the skin issues got a little better. However, my hormones were still out of balance, and a year of strict dieting had led me to an unhealthy relationship with food. I knew that what I was doing was not working, but I was not willing to give up. I was determined to find a way to fuel my body—to not only support my active lifestyle and help me accomplish my physical goals, but also to allow me to be as healthy as possible and at the same time honor my core beliefs. That's how the Plant-Powered Diet was born.

I have dedicated the past 23 years of personal studies to understanding how the body works and how to make it perform at its best. What I have found over and over again is that living plant-based foods are pure medicine for the body, mind and spirit. Whether you're a competitive athlete, weekend warrior or someone who simply wants to feel and perform better in the gym, at work or at home, switching to a diet centered on fresh fruits, vegetables, herbs, nuts, seeds and whole grains can have a profoundly positive impact not only on your health and performance but also on the environment. The Plant-Powered Diet creates a shift in the way we think, feel, behave and interact with our planet. To me, that's a win-win situation. Wouldn't you agree?

I am grateful for this opportunity to share my 20-plus-year journey as a plant-based athlete, fitness coach, vegan chef and yogi with you. It's nice to know that you are out there, reading these words, improving your life in one way or another and perhaps learning something from my experience. I am not expecting everyone to agree with everything in this book, but if even one of its readers gets a little higher, healthier and happier, then I would write this again a thousand times over. I hope you enjoy the read.

## What You Can Expect from This Book

This book is designed to help you attain the next level of vitality, to overcome the myths and misconceptions that stand in your way of building a lean, muscular body capable of endless energy and stamina.

In the following pages, I will outline the concept of the Plant-Powered Diet, offer practical ways and examples of how you can make this lifestyle work for you and provide you with more than 80 recipes to fuel your performance. I suggest here that for this approach to be effective, you should first adopt a positive attitude that a plant-based lifestyle can and will work for you. My second piece of advice is that you educate yourself on the power of whole, living plant-based foods. Start with reading the sections in this book that precede the recipes. However, don't stop there. Keep learning. Refer to the resources section (page 216) for literature and material that will help you grow further.

Finally, have fun while you embark on this journey. There may be some ups and downs while your body adjusts and adapts to new foods. Depending on your previous lifestyle, you may experience anything from cold- and flu-like symptoms to some major or minor muscle and joint pains. These are all gifts; your body is detoxing and working its magic. During these initial stages of your plant-powered journey, you can carry on with your regular fitness routine. Keep in mind, though, that you may not feel as strong during your workouts and may get lightheaded at times. Trust that soon these symptoms will pass and you will have more energy, mental clarity, strength and endurance than ever before.

And now it's my joy to share the Plant-Powered experience with you!

With love & light,

# core principles

## Getting Started: General Guidelines

**Came from a plant, eat it;
was made in a plant, don't.
—Michael Pollan**

Start by thinking of your plant-based journey as "an abundant lifestyle." Focus your attention on the things that you are adding rather than the things you are taking away. It's our human nature to avoid pain, so by choosing to focus on the lack, you will create suffering, and it will be quite challenging to change your old habits.

Here are some general guidelines for you to keep in mind as you begin your new living plant-based diet:

- Nourish your body with clean, whole, natural foods and avoid refined, processed and junk foods.
- Choose organic and local whenever possible.
- Eat produce that is in season (see the resources section on page 216).
- Eat real food, rather than relying on supplements.
- Drink fresh juice each day.
- Stay hydrated.
- Eat foods you enjoy and that agree with you.
- Eat until satisfied; do not overeat.

## The Plant-Powered Foods

No matter if you are a professional athlete or someone who is looking to reach higher physical and mental health—a combination of the following foods should be the core of your diet.

## Vegetables

Green leafy vegetables, such as romaine lettuce, dinosaur kale, collards, Swiss chard, spinach and microgreens, are some of the most nutrient-rich foods. They provide an excellent source of calcium, iron, phytonutrients and high-quality proteins. Furthermore, they are alkaline-forming and full of active enzymes. To build strength and muscle, recover faster, improve your performance and reach high levels of health and fitness, include a large green leafy salad into your diet every day.

In-season colorful veggies offer an amazing array of health benefits.

Red and yellow bell peppers, beets, carrots, purple cabbage, tomatoes—all of these colors mean you are getting a wider array of health-promoting antioxidants that are linked with better blood sugar management, less inflammation and healthier skin and eyesight.

## LEAFY GREENS

Try all kinds of greens, find those that you enjoy the most and make sure to include them into your diet daily.

| | | |
|---|---|---|
| ARUGULA | DANDELION GREENS | MICROGREENS |
| BABY SPINACH | DINOSAUR KALE | PARSLEY |
| BEET GREENS | ENDIVE | ROMAINE LETTUCE |
| BOK CHOY | FRISÉE | SWISS CHARD |
| BUTTER LETTUCE | LEAFY SPROUTS (SUCH AS ALFALFA, RADISH, BROCCOLI, CLOVER, ETC.) | WATERCRESS |
| CILANTRO | | |
| COLLARD GREENS | | |

# IN-SEASON COLORFUL VEGGIES

Consume a variety of in-season, preferably local and organic veggies daily to help improve your vitality and overall quality of your life. Some of our all-time favorites include:

| | | |
|---|---|---|
| BEETS | CUCUMBERS | PURPLE CABBAGE |
| BELL PEPPERS | FRESH GINGER | RADISHES |
| BROCCOLI | GARLIC | TOMATOES |
| CARROTS | JALAPEÑO PEPPERS | ZUCCHINI |
| CAULIFLOWER | MUSHROOMS | |
| CELERY | ONIONS | |

As much as possible, eat these vegetables in their raw state to preserve the antioxidants and phytonutrients—both are very beneficial to your health and athletic performance.

# SEA VEGETABLES

For optimum health benefits, enjoy sea vegetables in regular but small amounts.

| | |
|---|---|
| DULSE | KOMBU |
| IRISH MOSS | NORI |
| KELP | WAKAME |

How to use them?

- Sprinkle dry seaweed on salads.
- Add dried kelp/dulse to smoothies, energy bars or workout drinks as a source of electrolytes.
- Incorporate into recipes (substitute kelp noodles for pasta, use sheets of nori as wraps or add to veggie soups for extra flavor).
- Replace table salt with kelp granules or ground dulse.

Sea vegetables are another nutrient-rich, alkaline-forming food group that should be included in your plant-powered diet. They are a great source of minerals and provide a respectable amount of easily digested chlorophyll and protein. Seaweed contains a concentrated source of iodine and an amino acid called tyrosine—both required for the thyroid gland to function correctly and also a natural way to replenish electrolytes lost during physical activity.

### Fruits

Raw fruits are, in many ways, our most natural food. They're alkaline-forming, easy to digest, satisfying and can be directly used by the body for energy, with a high rate of efficiency.

Try to include several pieces of fresh fruit in your diet daily. Aim for ripe and nonhybridized fruit (those that contain seeds). It is also best to consume locally grown organic fruits during their season.

For ideal digestion, eat preferably one kind of fruit at a time. Since fruits leave the stomach within 20 to 40 minutes, it is better not to eat them with other foods, which could lead to fermentation, bloating and even diarrhea. The best times for eating fruit are midmorning and midafternoon, or for breakfast with nothing else.

### Fats

Fat is probably the most misunderstood macronutrient. Raw plant fats are essential to our health—they provide energy, protect the wall of each cell in the body and help lubricate the joints as well as the digestive tract. Many raw nuts and seeds contain omega-3 and omega-6 essential fatty acids (EFAs). These essential fats support the function of the cardiovascular, immune and nervous systems, as well as encourage proper absorption of certain nutrients. For an athlete, these fats play an important role in repair and recovery, helping reduce inflammation in the body. Getting enough of these healthy fats through what you eat is essential for long-term athletic performance.

## HI-ENERGY FRUITS

It is also best to consume locally grown, organic fruits during their season.*

APPLES

APRICOTS

AVOCADOS

BANANAS

BERRIES (ALL KINDS)

CHERRIES

DATES

FIGS

GRAPEFRUIT

GRAPES

LEMONS

LIMES

MANGOES

MELONS (ALL KINDS WITH SEEDS)

OLIVES (RAW)

ORANGES

PAPAYA

PEACHES

PEARS

PINEAPPLE

PLANTAINS

PLUMS

PRUNES

RAISINS

POMEGRANATES

YOUNG COCONUTS

*seasonal produce guide available at activevegetarian.com

# RAW PLANT FATS

AVOCADOS

COCONUT (MEAT, MILK, BUTTER/MANNA)

RAW OLIVES

**RAW NUTS:**

ALMONDS

BRAZIL NUTS

CASHEWS

HAZELNUTS

MACADAMIA NUTS

PECANS

PISTACHIOS

WALNUTS

**RAW SEEDS:**

CHIA SEEDS

FLAXSEEDS

HEMP HEARTS

POPPY SEEDS

PUMPKIN SEEDS

SESAME SEEDS

SUNFLOWER SEEDS

**RAW/COLD-PRESSED/ EXTRA-VIRGIN OILS (LITTLE GOES A LONG WAY):**

COCONUT OIL

FLAXSEED OIL

HEMP SEED OIL

OLIVE OIL

Always be sure to choose raw/cold-pressed/extra virgin oils instead of refined versions which may be partly or fully hydrogenated, therefore being stripped of any positive health effects.

Coconut oil is the only fat you'll want to use for cooking with heat—that's because it's one of the only oils that can be heated to high temperatures without being converted into unhealthy trans fats.

## Complex Unrefined Carbohydrates

Carbohydrates are our body's first choice for fuel, and it's important to include them in our plant-powered diet. The challenge is that over 90 percent of the carbs consumed by most people today are highly refined, highly processed and mostly in the form of white flour and sugar. If your goal is to enjoy excellent health and perform well physically and mentally, then we encourage you to stay away from them! Personally, we get almost all of our carbohydrates from fruit, which is a simple carbohydrate that requires less work for the body to break down. Once in a while, we include complex carbohydrates from sprouted whole grains, pseudograins, pulses and starchy vegetables. Let's take a closer look at each of these.

Sprouted whole grains are rich in protein, satisfying and offer some essential macronutrients, including the B vitamins (such as folate), vitamin C, iron and essential amino acids often lacking in grains, such as lysine.

Another benefit of sprouted grains is the fiber content that helps keep blood sugar levels in check and deliver slow-release, steady energy to support your active lifestyle throughout the day.

Pseudograins are not grains in the classic sense; they are seeds, often used in place of conventional grains. Since pseudograins are gluten-free, they are easily digestible and suitable for those who are gluten intolerant or sensitive to gluten. Other than being a beneficial source of complex carbohydrate, pseudograins also provide high-quality protein, zinc and B vitamins.

Pulses are part of the legume family (any plants that grow in pods), but the term pulse refers only to the dried, edible seeds within the pod. Beans, lentils, chickpeas and split peas are the most common types of pulses. Pulses are unique because they have distinct health benefits apart from other legumes. Unlike such legumes as peanuts and soy, for example, pulses are low in fat and very high in protein and fiber.

## SPROUTED WHOLE GRAINS

Sprouted grains are often eaten raw, lightly cooked or ground into flour. They are a great addition to salads, Nourish Bowls (page 146) and homemade breads.

| | | |
|---|---|---|
| BARLEY | OATS | RYE |
| KAMUT | RICE | SPELT |
| | | TEFF |

If you choose to eat baked goods, such as bread and tortilla wraps, be sure to eat those that are made from whole sprouted grains.

# PSEUDOGRAINS

Due to their high fiber and antioxidant content, all these "grains" are beneficial for blood sugar control, making them a great "comfort" food to eat with your evening meal or as a part of your postworkout meal.

| | | |
|---|---|---|
| AMARANTH | MILLET | WILD RICE |
| BUCKWHEAT | QUINOA | |

# PULSES

Due to the high fiber content, it's best to consume these after your training session. You'll get a number of vitamins, minerals and antioxidants to maintain your health, immunity and proper recovery.

| **LENTILS:** | **DRIED PEAS:** | BLACK-EYED PEAS |
|---|---|---|
| BLACK | GREEN | CHICKPEAS (GARBANZO BEANS) |
| GREEN | YELLOW | |
| FRENCH GREEN | **BEANS:** | FAVA |
| RED | ADZUKI | KIDNEY |
| SMALL BROWN | BLACK BEANS | NAVY |
| | | PINTO |

Pulses are cost effective and can be used in many ways. Add a scoop of lentils, beans or chickpeas to a salad or Nourish Bowl (page 146), make a dip for veggies or a sandwich with hummus.

We suggest soaking and/or sprouting pulses before using. If you choose to buy canned rather than dried pulses, make sure to rinse them well.

## STARCHY VEGETABLES

These whole plant-based foods are rich in fiber and they take longer to break down during digestion. They provide a controlled release of energy throughout the day, rather than a huge spike and subsequent drop.

| | | |
|---|---|---|
| CORN | PUMPKIN | WINTER SQUASH |
| GREEN PEAS | SWEET POTATOES | YAMS |

## SUPERFOODS

Here we are listing some of our favorite superfoods. We encourage you to stick to organic and fair trade–certified products, whenever possible. You can find a list of ethical, fair trade–certified companies in the resources section on page 216.

| | | |
|---|---|---|
| AÇAÍ BERRIES | CHLORELLA | MAQUI POWDER |
| ALOE VERA | GOLDEN BERRIES | MULBERRIES |
| ASHWAGANDHA | GOJI BERRIES | SPIRULINA |
| CACAO | LUCUMA POWDER | WHEATGRASS |
| CAMU CAMU POWDER | MACA | |

Superfoods can be used as an ingredient in smoothies, juices, nut mylks, salads, power bars, energy snacks and even desserts!

## Starchy Vegetables

Starchy vegetables are an important part of the Plant-Powered Diet; however, only modest amounts are needed.

## Superfoods

What makes a food super?

A superfood is a food that is more nutrient rich than regular food and has unique health-promoting properties. These foods typically contain higher levels of vitamins, minerals, antioxidants and some even contain amino acids, adaptogens and chlorophyll. Certain superfoods have medicinal properties as well, from treating seasonal allergies to regulating hormones. The benefit of including superfoods in your plant-powered diet is that you will be getting an impressive amount of nutrition and consume much less food. Therefore, superfoods are especially beneficial for those with weight-loss goals, as well as for anyone with a weakened or impaired immune or digestive system. Since the intent of the Plant-Powered Diet is to eat the most natural and nutrient-rich foods, we feel that every single person can benefit from incorporating some superfoods into their daily regime.

## Fermented Foods

Fermented, a.k.a. cultured foods, are known to help "heal and seal" your gut which will get you on your way towards optimal health. You can't rely on cultured foods alone; however, they can be a beneficial addition to your plant-powered diet. So, what exactly is fermented food? Fermentation is the process of culturing healthy bacteria in food. Cultured foods, such as coconut yogurt, sauerkraut, raw cultured veggies and kombucha, are rich sources of probiotics and enzymes that help support the immune system and fight inflammation in the body. Eating raw fermented foods and drinks, preferably before or with every meal in some form, essentially improves the quality of the whole meal and allows for better digestion as well as absorption.

Fermented foods are alive and active, full of enzymes and billions of life-giving microorganisms. Once in the belly, those bacterial armies get to work, helping to balance your gut bacteria and stomach acids. They also release enzymes to help ease and improve digestion, enhance elimination, balance unhealthy levels of candida and increase nutrient absorption overall.

**Plant-Powered Fermented Foods**

- Coconut yogurt (page 55)
- Cultured nut cheese, such as Almond Ricotta (page 203)
- Sauerkraut (page 67)
- Raw cultured vegetables
- Kimchi
- Kombucha
- Kefir, made with water, coconut water or plant-based milks
- Tempeh
- Miso (unpasteurized)
- Natto

Our approach is to have a serving (a spoonful or small glass) of fermented food before a meal or a snack (if possible). Making your own fermented foods is easy and inexpensive—for more information on this topic, see the resources section on page 216.

## Protein: How to Get Enough

As I enter my 23rd year on a plant-based journey, I get very passionate about the question "But where do you get your protein?" I find it to be an exciting teaching opportunity. From my experience, the word protein is incredibly misunderstood. In our Western world, we have been conditioned to believe that meat = protein. Therefore, it's no wonder that when we talk about plant-based diets, usually the most important question people have is "How can I get enough protein?"

For those of us who are active and work out regularly, the subject of protein is even more prevalent. You might worry that when you stop eating meat, you'll get too thin. You'll lose all of your hard-earned muscles, and you may even lose your hair. Your performance will suffer, you won't have enough energy, you will get sick or weak, and so on.

# FUNCTION OF PROTEIN

Proteins are an important component of every cell in the body.

It produces antibodies for the immune system.

It produces enzymes that are required for many chemical reactions in the body (digestion, absorption and blood coagulation).

Dietary protein is important for the proper growth of all cells and in building and reconstructing body tissue in muscles, body organs, eyes, hair and skin.

Protein also contributes to the formation of antibodies, hemoglobin and hormones, and helps maintain proper electrolyte balance in the body.

Protein is a source of fuel when muscle glycogen levels are low (during prolonged, intense training).

If you're concerned about your protein intake and interested in the healthiest way to get enough through plant-based foods, please keep reading.

### What Is Protein?

Protein is an essential nutrient that plays a crucial role in our overall health and well-being. It is throughout the body—in muscle, bone, skin, hair and virtually every other body part or tissue. Protein molecules consist of 20-plus basic building blocks called amino acids, which are made available to the body through the process of digestion. There are two categories of amino acids: essential and nonessential. Essential amino acids have to be consumed through the diet, as our body cannot produce them. Nonessential amino acids are created in our body from the food we consume.

### Animal vs. Plant-Based Protein

Plant-based diets get accused of lacking the complete proteins required daily by the human body. Although it is known that all essential amino acids can be obtained from plant-based foods, meat as a source of protein is still considered to be the better option.

So, how can we get in shape without animal protein?

I would suggest we look at the strongest animals on the planet—elephants, gorillas, wild horses. How do they get their protein? (They are all vegan.) We are not the same as these amazing, strong creatures; however, over the years, it has been proven that we do not need to depend on eating animal proteins to fulfill our daily needs. We can live and perform perfectly well without meat, fish, dairy or eggs as long as we have a properly balanced diet, clean liver and healthy gut.

To understand the animal-versus-plant-protein argument in more depth, we need to look at the digestive process of protein that happens predominantly in the stomach and small intestine. Stomach acid separates protein into smaller basic units of amino acids. The amino acids then travel to the small intestine, where they get absorbed into the blood for delivery to the body's cells. The liver is a key regulator of the body's amino acid pool and will direct what happens with incoming amino acids. In some instances, the protein will serve as an energy source and aid in muscle repair; at other times, it will be stored in the amino acid pool of the body until it's required to make additional proteins.

A common misconception about plant-based diets is that they don't provide enough protein. That is not the case if you eat a plant-based whole food diet. Such foods as pseudograins, amaranth, quinoa, buckwheat and wild rice are all around 20 percent protein. Spinach and kale are 45 percent protein. Spirulina and chlorella are around 65 percent protein. When you eat a variety of plant-based foods, you're going to get enough protein. Plus, eating plant-based proteins is far better for the environment as these foods require fewer natural resources to produce. Also, when you switch to a plant-based diet, you are eating lower on the food chain and therefore not taking in as many herbicides, pesticides and hormones. In addition, plant-based whole foods are easier to digest and alkaline-forming, which means they reduce inflammation; in addition, they're good for bone health.

As far as I know, there is no scientific evidence as yet that would indicate a protein deficiency in those who never eat animal protein. On the contrary, as a society, we may not be suffering from lack of protein at all, but from its overconsumption. By filling up the connective tissues of our body with unused protein, we turn the body into an overflowing pool of harmful acids and waste, thereby laying a fertile ground for such diseases as osteoporosis, heart disease, rheumatoid arthritis and cancer.

The root of the problem lies in our body's inability to break down meat protein into amino acids properly. Chunks of undigested meat pass into the intestinal tract, and along with them, parasites. Most of these parasites are vigorous suckers that can survive the heat applied during cooking, as well as the human stomach acid. Carnivorous animals, on the other hand, kill these parasites instantly while passing them through the stomach. Their stomachs produce 20 times more hydrochloric acid than ours does. This massive amount of acid helps the animals break down the meat proteins into their essential components.

As you can see now, the main digestive work in carnivorous animals takes place in their stomach and not in the small intestine (as occurs in humans). The meat stays in their relatively short intestinal tract for only a little while. Our small intestine, which is 16 to 20 feet (5 to 6 m) long, processes most natural foods within a matter of several hours. However, meat may stay in our small intestine for up to 20 to 48 hours, by which time much of it is putrefied or decayed. The

rotting process results in the formation of poisonous toxins. These poisons begin to act as disease-causing agents in the body. It's not unusual for the "leftovers" of undigested meat to linger in the large intestinal walls of humans for 20 to 30 years or longer.

For our health as well as that of our planet, there isn't a better choice than a diet of whole, organic, plant-based living foods.

## The Protein Combining Myth

"Protein combining," a diet trend that became popular in the 1970s, was based on the misconception that vegan diets provide insufficient amino acids. The concept was that we needed to eat so-called complementary proteins together (for example, rice and beans) to make up for their relative shortfalls. However, this misconception was proven wrong decades ago. To be clear, a "complete protein" is a protein that contains all nine of the essential amino acids our body needs to function: histidine, isoleucine, leucine, lysine, methionine, phenylalanine, threonine, tryptophan and valine. Those amino acids are "essential," but our body can't make them, so they must be derived from the foods we eat. While it's true that some plant proteins are relatively low in certain essential amino acids, our body knows how to make up for it. Studies show that our body can combine complementary proteins eaten within 24 hours. When protein is consumed and broken down into different amino acids, an overall "amino acid pool" is formed via which we pull from to build protein in the body. Simply put, when eating a variety of whole plant foods, you can easily acquire all the essential amino acids, and you don't need to worry about pairing foods to create "complete proteins." We recycle about 90 grams of protein per day, so our body can mix and match amino acids based on what we need.

## Protein and Muscle

Another big misconception about a plant-based diet is that you can't build muscle. Many fitness "experts" argue that you need to consume lots of protein, preferably animal protein, to notice significant muscle gain. That's simply an incorrect assumption. Plant-based proteins can provide the same complete proteins as the traditional animal-based muscle-building protein sources, and as a plant-powered athlete, you can build incredible muscle bulk as well as strength. Of course, you do have to engage in regular weightlifting exercises. Read more at "Lean Muscle Building" (page 35).

# HIGH-QUALITY PLANT-BASED PROTEIN SOURCES

## VEGETABLES

| INGREDIENT | AMOUNT | PROTEIN (grams) |
|---|---|---|
| Spinach | 1 cup (30 g), cooked | 5.4 |
| Corn | 1 large cob | 5 |
| Collard Greens | 1 cup (36 g), cooked | 5 |
| Asparagus | 1 cup (134 g), cooked | 4.3 |
| Sweet Potato | 1 medium | 4 |
| Brussels Sprouts | 1 cup (38 g), cooked | 3.9 |
| Broccoli | 1 cup (71 g), cooked | 3.7 |
| Dulse, Dried | 2 tbsp (6 g) | 3.6 |
| Mustard Greens | 1 cup (56 g), cooked | 3.6 |
| Swiss Chard | 1 cup (36 g), cooked | 3.3 |
| Beets | 1 cup (136 g) | 2.9 |
| Mushrooms, Oyster | 1 cup (86 g), cooked | 2.8 |
| Kale | 1 cup (67 g), cooked | 2.5 |
| Green Beans | 1 cup (110 g), cooked | 2.4 |
| Cauliflower | 1 cup (100 g), cooked | 2.3 |
| Mushrooms, Shiitake | 1 cup (97 g), cooked | 2.3 |
| Squash, Winter | 1 cup (140 g), cooked | 1.8 |
| Squash, Summer | 1 cup (124 g), cooked | 1.6 |
| Turnip Greens | 1 cup (38 g), cooked | 1.6 |
| Tomato | 1 cup (180 g), raw | 1.6 |
| Carrots | 1 cup (128 g), raw | 1.1 |
| Olives, Black | 1 cup (180 g) | 1.1 |
| Wheatgrass, Juice | 2 oz (60 ml) | 1 |
| Bell Peppers | 1 cup (124 g), raw | 0.9 |
| Celery | 1 cup (101 g), raw | 0.7 |
| Cucumber | 1 cup (104 g), raw | 0.7 |
| Lettuce, Romaine | 1 cup (47 g), raw | 0.6 |

## FRESH FRUIT

| INGREDIENT | AMOUNT | PROTEIN (grams) |
|---|---|---|
| Cherimoya | 1 medium | 7 |
| Sapote | 1 medium | 5 |
| Passion Fruit | 1 cup (236 g) | 5 |
| Pomegranate | 1 medium | 4.7 |
| Guava | 1 cup (165 g) | 4.2 |

| INGREDIENT | AMOUNT | PROTEIN (grams) |
|---|---|---|
| Avocado | 1 medium | 4 |
| Durian | 1 cup (243 g) | 4 |
| Jackfruit | 1 cup (165 g) | 2.8 |
| Blackberries | 1 cup (144 g) | 2 |
| Grapefruit | 1 medium | 1.6 |
| Raspberries | 1 cup (123 g) | 1.5 |
| Peach | 1 medium | 1.4 |
| Mango | 1 cup (165 g) | 1.4 |
| Cantaloupe | 1 cup (160 g) | 1.3 |
| Papaya | 1 medium | 1.3 |
| Banana | 1 medium | 1.3 |
| Orange | 1 medium | 1.2 |
| Figs | 3 medium | 1.2 |
| Blueberries | 1 cup (148 g) | 1.1 |
| Grapes | 1 cup (151 g) | 1.1 |
| Strawberries | 1 cup (144 g) | 1 |
| Watermelon | 1 cup (152 g) | 0.9 |
| Pineapple | 1 cup (165 g) | 0.9 |
| Kiwi | 1 medium | 0.8 |
| Pear | 1 medium | 0.6 |
| Lemon/Lime | 1 medium | 0.6 |
| Apricot | 1 medium | 0.5 |
| Apple | 1 medium | 0.5 |
| Plum | 1 medium | 0.5 |

**DRIED FRUIT**

| INGREDIENT | AMOUNT | PROTEIN (grams) |
|---|---|---|
| Goji Berries | 1 cup (111 g) | 15 |
| Mulberries, White | 1 cup (120 g) | 12 |
| Goldenberries | 1 cup (112 g) | 12 |
| Raisins | 1 cup (165 g) | 5 |
| Figs | 1 cup (149 g) | 5 |
| Apricots | 1 cup (130 g) | 4.4 |
| Dates | 1 cup (147 g) | 4.4 |
| Prunes | 1 cup (174 g) | 3.9 |

## ALGAE

| INGREDIENT | AMOUNT | PROTEIN (grams) |
| --- | --- | --- |
| Chlorella | 1 tbsp (9 g) | 3.8 |
| Spirulina | 1 tbsp (7 g) | 4 |

## NUTS & SEEDS

| INGREDIENT | AMOUNT | PROTEIN (grams) |
| --- | --- | --- |
| Chia Seeds | ¼ cup (40 g) | 12 |
| Hemp Seeds | ¼ cup (40 g) | 10 |
| Flaxseeds | ¼ cup (42 g) | 8 |
| Sunflower Seeds | ¼ cup (35 g) | 8 |
| Almonds | ¼ cup (36 g) | 7 |
| Pumpkin Seeds | ¼ cup (30 g) | 7 |
| Sesame Seeds | ¼ cup (36 g) | 7 |
| Pistachios | ¼ cup (31 g) | 6 |
| Walnuts | ¼ cup (25 g) | 5 |
| Brazil Nuts | ¼ cup (33 g) | 5 |
| Hazelnuts | ¼ cup (34 g) | 5 |
| Pine Nuts | ¼ cup (34 g) | 4 |
| Cashews | ¼ cup (37 g) | 4 |

## LEGUMES

| INGREDIENT | AMOUNT | PROTEIN (grams) |
| --- | --- | --- |
| Lentils | 1 cup (256 g) | 18 |
| Adzuki | 1 cup (197 g) | 18 |
| White Beans | 1 cup (202 g) | 17 |
| Navy Beans | 1 cup (208 g) | 16 |
| Split Peas | 1 cup (197 g) | 16 |
| Black Beans | 1 cup (194 g) | 15 |
| Garbanzo Beans (Chickpeas) | 1 cup (200 g) | 15 |
| Kidney Beans | 1 cup (184 g) | 15 |
| Great Northern Beans | 1 cup (183 g) | 15 |
| Lima Beans | 1 cup (164 g) | 15 |
| Black-Eyed Peas | 1 cup (145 g) | 14 |
| Mung Beans | 1 cup (207 g) | 14 |
| Pinto Beans | 1 cup (193 g) | 14 |
| Green Peas | 1 cup (145 g) | 9 |

## GRAINS (COOKED)

| INGREDIENT | AMOUNT | PROTEIN (grams) |
| --- | --- | --- |
| Spelt* | 1 cup (194 g) | 11 |
| Black Rice | 1 cup (158 g) | 10 |
| Teff | 1 cup (252 g) | 9.5 |
| Amaranth | 1 cup (246 g) | 9.4 |
| Quinoa | 1 cup (185 g) | 8 |
| Wild Rice | 1 cup (164 g) | 7 |
| Millet | 1 cup (174 g) | 6.1 |
| Oat Groats | 1 cup (168 g) | 6 |
| Buckwheat | 1 cup (168 g) | 5.7 |
| Brown Rice | 1 cup (195 g) | 5 |

*contains gluten

## MORE REASONS TO EAT RAW FOODS

- Increased energy & stamina
- Detox & cleanse
- Weight loss
- Slow down the aging process
- Mental clarity & focus
- Improved digestion
- Disease prevention

- Heart health
- Faster recovery
- Stronger immune function
- Decreased cravings
- Emotional & spiritual balance
- Smaller carbon footprint

## Benefits of Raw Foods

The Plant-Powered Diet is centered on living plant food with a significant emphasis on raw food that has not been heated above 115°F (46°C). Over the years, we found that by including more of these foods into our daily meal plan, we have been able to improve our health and enhance our performance dramatically. How is that possible? Well, it's simple—by eating more raw plant food in its purest form, which contains all the enzymes, nutrients and minerals that give us more strength, endurance, energy and vitality, our body can take maximum nutritional benefit from it.

When food gets heated above 115°F (46°C) for an extended period, the enzymes in the food are destroyed or denatured and are therefore unable to provide the same nutritional value. When you predominantly consume foods that do not have enzymes present, your body must strain to work overtime to digest the food. If your body is working overtime with digestion, it has less time to focus on other bodily processes. As a result, you are exhausting your physical energies, increasing risks of illness and injury, decreasing nutrient absorption and increasing inflammation.

Being aware of this is especially important if you're looking to improve your health and athletic performance. If you don't always burden your body with digesting and assimilating hard-to-digest foods—such as processed foods and cooked animal protein—it has more energy to increase recovery and healing. Does it mean that you should eat only raw foods? No, you do not have to. However, it is wise to eat more raw and less cooked, and that's why Nikki and I are on a mission to help you find simple, everyday ways to incorporate raw foods into your diet.

## Alkalinity

There's another part of this puzzle: alkalinity. Our body strives to maintain a particular pH level, which is a measure of the acidity or alkalinity of our blood. Levels of pH can range from 0 (very acidic) up to 14 (highly alkaline). The human body is designed to operate within a very narrow pH range, around 7.365, which is slightly alkaline. If our pH drops, our body becomes too acidic and we are more susceptible to chronic disease. It's important to understand that cancer cells and disease thrive in acidic, low-oxygen environments. Throw them into an alkaline environment rich in oxygen, and they'll never be able to survive.

So, how do we get more alkaline? You guessed right: Eat more raw foods. Maintaining an acid/alkaline balance in your diet is one of the most influential ways to prevent disease and improve performance as an athlete. Fresh raw veggies, greens, fruits, sprouted grains, nuts and seeds, vegetable juices and algae are heavily alkaline. They help our body stay in a healthy pH range, minimize stress, help reduce inflammation (making your muscles more efficient) and support long-term wellness. With a few exceptions, those same foods (veggies, fruits, algae) are also alkaline when cooked healthily. However, if you eat them raw, you get the alkalinity as well as the rich nutrient value. A winning combination!

## Why Juice?

You and you alone are responsible for the outcome of your diet. Nourishment from foods largely influences your health, performance and even your state of mind. Your body is composed of billions of microscopic cells. Cells are the fundamental units of life, "the bricks" from which all your tissues and organs are made. Since disease originates at a cellular level, the health of single cells is what creates a healthy body. Healthy cells produce healthy tissues. Healthy tissues form healthy organs, including the heart and brain. Healthy organs create healthy systems, such as the immune system, and healthy systems make a healthy body.

Fruits, vegetables and their juices are packed with vitamins, minerals and a whole host of other essential nutrients needed for optimum health. It's the juices held within the fiber of fresh fruits and vegetables that feed the body by nourishing every cell and helping to flush the system of waste.

Several years ago, Nikki and I committed ourselves to the Daily Juicing Habit. We can honestly tell you that the power of juicing is real. If you've never experienced it, you are in for a treat. We sincerely believe that this single habit of drinking a big glass of freshly made organic juice each day can change your life. We've never had one person come back to us after developing the Daily Juicing Habit and say they felt worse than before. This stuff works!

# ALKALINE & ACID FORMING FOODS

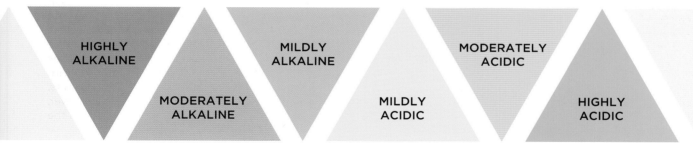

HIGHLY ALKALINE — MODERATELY ALKALINE — MILDLY ALKALINE — MILDLY ACIDIC — MODERATELY ACIDIC — HIGHLY ACIDIC

**EAT MORE**            **EAT LESS**

| | | | | | |
|---|---|---|---|---|---|
| 9.0 + alkaline water | watermelon & most other melons | apples | green bananas | chocolate | coffee |
| | | oranges | plums | | black tea |
| | mangoes | bananas | dried fruits | chickpeas | sweetened fruits |
| Himalayan and sea salt | blackberries | blueberries | | lima beans | |
| | raspberries | strawberries | Brazil nuts, pecans, hazelnuts & most other nuts | white rice | pasteurized juices |
| lemons | fresh dates | cranberries | | white & whole wheat | |
| limes | fresh figs | coconut | | | |
| | grapefruits | | most legumes | | sodas |
| cucumbers | | mushrooms | | ocean fish | alcohol |
| celery | avocados | cauliflower | amaranth | | |
| Brussels sprouts | tomatoes | zucchini | millet | most microwaved food | artificial sweeteners |
| broccoli | bell peppers | chives | oats | | white sugar |
| asparagus | beets | leeks | barley | | refined flours |
| Swiss chard | green beans | most herbs & spices | rye & most other grains | most bottled waters and sports drinks | processed grains |
| mustard greens | okra | | | | processed foods |
| parsley | radishes | buckwheat | | | fried foods |
| kale | red onions | quinoa | rice milk | | |
| | endives | most sprouted grains | soy milk | ketchup | |
| fermented vegetables | arugula | lentils | almond milk | mustard | pasteurized dairy |
| raw vegetable juices | ginger | soybeans | sunflower oil | most pharmaceutical drugs | animal meat |
| | garlic | tofu | grape seed oil | | eggs |
| chlorella, kelp & other sea vegetables | sweet potatoes | | canola oil | | shellfish |
| | carrots | flax oil | corn oil | iodized table salt | |
| | most lettuces | avocado oil | honey | | |
| wheatgrass & most young grasses | | coconut oil | maple syrup | | |
| | pumpkin seeds | | molasses | | |
| sprouts | almonds | | | | |
| | | | freshwater fish | | |
| | olive oil | | | | |

Good news . . . pleasure, laughter, happiness, rest and sleep are all ALKALINE forming!

Juicing is a process that extracts water and nutrients from produce and discards the fiber. Without the fiber, the digestive system doesn't have to work as hard to break down the food and can absorb the nutrients. It makes the nutrients more readily available to the body in much larger quantities. The result is a "liquid meal" that is a very concentrated source of enzymes and micronutrients—vitamins, minerals, antioxidants and phytochemicals.

Juicing also helps you consume multiple servings of fruits and vegetables and deliver far more health-promoting nutrients to your system than you would by eating them straight or preparing them in any other way. It would be challenging to chew several pounds of raw carrots in a day, but when they are squeezed into a juice, you can deliver enormous amounts of vitamin A to improve your night vision, acquire healthy skin and detoxify your liver. A clean liver efficiently processes all the chemicals we expose ourselves to daily. The liver is your fat-burning organ, and when the liver is clean, you will lose excess fat if you need to.

## But What about the Fiber?
Great question. The answer is simple: Most whole fruits and vegetables require many hours of digesting to provide nourishment to the cells and tissues of your body. Although the fibers have practically no nourishing value, they do play an essential role in cleaning up the intestines, and therefore we do need to eat whole fruits and vegetables in addition to drinking juices. However, the removal of the fibers during juicing enables juices to be quickly digested and assimilated, sometimes in a matter of minutes, with a minimum of effort and stress on your digestive system.

## Isn't Juice High in Sugar?
Another common concern is ingesting too much sugar. If you make your juices mostly from fruits—and yes, they do taste delicious—then your sugar intake is most likely much higher than it should be. If you have diabetes or problems with your blood sugar, you need to be aware of this and be careful. However, this is easy to fix. Always make sure that the foundation of your juice is vegetable-based with many green leaves and only add fruits (or just one fruit) as flavor enhancers to make it fruity and tasty.

## What Can I Juice?
While carrots, apples, oranges, grapes and pineapple are superdelicious, don't forget about herbs (parsley, cilantro, mint and fennel) and bitter veggies (dandelion leaves, watercress and arugula), which can add both flavor and extra nutrients. Lemon and lime add a fresh zing and plenty of vitamin C. Traditionally, ginger is used to ease digestive discomfort and reduce inflammation; add a small cube of ginger for a little bite to your morning juice. Jalapeño pepper, turmeric and cayenne pepper also make delicious and medicinal additions.

Try adding purple cabbage to your carrots when juicing. Cabbage helps protect your body from cancer, boosts your body's detoxification enzymes and removes environmental estrogens, which can create a variety of hormone problems and stubborn belly fat.

Juiced greens, such as spinach, kale, collards and parsley, are superbeneficial in your plant-based diet because they add a lot of chlorophyll, which is a powerful blood cleanser and blood builder. Chlorophyll has a similar structure to human red blood cells, and adding many raw (uncooked) greens into your diet will deliver the building materials required for the body to produce much fresh blood. You will notice that your endurance and performance will increase after adding many raw greens.

Try to drink your juice right away. After fifteen minutes, light and air will destroy much of the nutrients. If you can't drink it immediately, transfer it to a dark, airtight container until you're ready.

Whenever possible, make your own fresh juice or buy a fresh one from a raw juice bar. Most store-bought and packaged juices are pasteurized, which makes them acid-forming, deprives them of natural enzymes and depletes the body of essential minerals and vitamins.

We encourage you to give the juicing habit an honest try. This simple practice of starting your day with a big glass of fresh juice is one significant step toward your athletic goal, health and longevity. If you would like more information on juicing and how to make it a daily habit, see the resources section on page 216.

## Soaking & Sprouting

Nuts, seeds, grains and beans are loaded with nutrients and especially popular with plant-based eaters as they offer a great source of protein. However, the high fiber content and natural agents that protect these foods can wreak havoc on our digestive system—ever felt bloated and gassy after eating beans? I can relate; the same thing used to happen to me. Not only did eating beans upset my stomach, but my mouth and throat would get itchy after eating certain nuts or seeds. Many people get serious digestive issues from these foods and assume they must eliminate them from their diet. For some, it might even become a reason they give up on plant-based eating altogether.

Barring the possibility of food sensitivities or allergies (in which case, you might have to eliminate them), there is a way to prepare nuts, seeds, grains and beans that makes them easier to digest. It might add some extra steps to your food prep. However, you will make your meals more digestible and avoid these uncomfortable reactions.

It turns out that all legumes, whole grains, most nuts and some seeds contain a variety of enzyme inhibitors, including phytic acid, that impair digestion. Phytic acid works by binding up minerals so they are unable to ignite the enzymatic reactions that tell a seed or nut to sprout until it is safe to do so. It's a protection that ensures the survival of the plant.

Nature allows the inhibitors and toxic substances to be removed easily when the conditions (enough rain and sunlight) are right. When it rains, the seed gets enough moisture so it can germinate and produce a plant. The plant then continues to grow with the sunlight. In the case of nuts, if an animal eats the nut, it could pass through the digestive system unharmed and possibly have a chance to sprout and grow a whole new plant.

Unfortunately, for humans, these inhibitors affect the digestion of these foods and do not allow us to fully absorb the minerals from them. Phytic acid is like a magnet for minerals, binding them up until the seed has started to germinate. We're talking essential minerals, such as calcium, magnesium, iron, zinc and copper.

By soaking and sprouting nuts, seeds, grains and beans, you are replicating nature's germination process of turning a seed into a plant. You can see it happening in front of your eyes! Mother Nature is incredible, isn't she?

The main benefits to soaking and sprouting are the ability to activate and multiply the nutrients, neutralize enzyme inhibitors and promote the growth of vital digestive enzymes.

This method is straightforward; the only thing that changes is the time it takes for the various items to germinate (see the charts on pages 28 and 29).

### Benefits of Soaking & Sprouting

**Soaking:**
- Reduces levels of water-soluble and heat-sensitive toxins and antinutrients, such as tannins, saponins, gluten, digestive enzyme inhibitors and lectins
- Reduces the flatulence factor
- Partially deactivates enzyme inhibitors
- Improves the digestibility and nutritional value of grains and legumes, and increases the enzymes
- Using sea salt in your soak water helps deactivate the enzyme inhibitors.

**Sprouting:**
- Activates food enzymes and increases the vitamin content
- Neutralizes antinutrients (enzyme inhibitors, tannins, phytic acid, lectin, gluten and other proteins)
- Enhances the nutrient bioavailability in grains

### How to Soak & Sprout

1. Rinse the nuts/seeds/grains/beans thoroughly and pour into a jar of roughly four times their volume (fill to the ¼ mark).
2. Fill the jar at least three-quarters full of water.
3. Soak overnight at room temperature. (We use our kitchen counter.)
4. In the morning, pour out the water from the nuts/seeds/grains/beans, then rinse with fresh water and strain.

# nut & seed SOAKING GUIDE

**MOST OTHER NUTS & SEEDS**
soak: 6–8 hrs

**ALMONDS**
soak: 8–12 hrs
salt per cup (143 g): 1 tsp
*sprout: 12 hrs*

**BRAZIL NUTS**
soak: 3–8 hrs
salt per cup (132 g): ½ tsp
*does not sprout*

**SUNFLOWER SEEDS**
soak: 6–8 hrs
salt per cup (120 g): 2 tsp (6 g)
*sprout: 1–2 days*

**CASHEWS**
soak: 2–6 hrs
salt per cup (148 g): 1 tsp
*does not sprout*

**PUMPKIN SEEDS**
soak: 6–8 hrs
salt per cup (120 g): 2 tsp (6 g)
*sprout: 1–2 days*

**HAZELNUTS**
soak: 8 hrs
salt per cup (136 g): 1 tsp
*does not sprout*

**WALNUTS**
soak: 4–7 hrs
salt per cup (100 g): ½ tsp
*does not sprout*

**MACADAMIAS**
soak: 7–12 hrs
salt per cup (134 g): 1 tsp
*does not sprout*

**PISTACHIOS**
soak: 6 hrs
salt per cup (124 g): ½ tsp
*does not sprout*

**PECANS**
soak: 4–6 hrs
salt per cup (100 g): ½ tsp
*does not sprout*

Using sea salt in your soaking water helps deactivate the enzyme inhibitors.

# seed, grain & legume
## SPROUTING GUIDE

**SESAME (UNHULLED)**
soak: 4–8 hrs
*sprout: 1–2 days*

**FLAX**
soak: 6 hrs
*sprout: 1–5 days*

**CHIA**
soak: 4 hrs
*sprout: 1–4 days*

**MUNG**
soak: 8 hrs
*sprout: 4–5 days*

**QUINOA**
soak: 3–4 hrs
*sprout: 2–3 days*

**PEA**
soak: 8 hrs
*sprout: 2–3 days*

**RICE**
soak: 8–12 hrs
*sprout: 2–3 days*

**ADZUKI**
soak: 8–12 hrs
*sprout: 3–5 days*

**AMARANTH**
soak: 3–5 hrs
*sprout: 3–5 days*

**GARBANZO**
soak: 12–48 hrs
*sprout: 2–4 days*

**KAMUT**
soak: 8–10 hrs
*sprout: 2–3 days*

**LENTIL**
soak: 8 hrs
*sprout: 2–3 days*

**MILLET**
soak: 5–8 hrs
*sprout: 1–2 days*

**RADISH**
soak: 6 hrs
*sprout: 3–5 days*

**OAT GROAT**
soak: 6–8 hrs
*sprout: 2–3 days*

**FENUGREEK**
soak: 6 hrs
*sprout: 2–5 days*

**ALFALFA**
soak: 8–12 hrs
*sprout: 3–5 days*

**CLOVER**
soak: 4–6 hrs
*sprout: 3–5 days*

**BUCKWHEAT (HULLED)**
soak: 6 hrs
*sprout: 1–2 days*

The steps on page 27 complete the soaking process. For sprouting, continue with the next steps.

1. Return the nuts/seeds/grains/beans to the jar.
2. Cover the jar with a cheesecloth and secure the cloth with a rubber band.
3. Briefly turn the jar upside down to drain the remaining water.
4. Place the jar on the kitchen counter on an angle (you want to be able to allow water to drain and airflow to enter), keep away from heat and allow some natural sunlight.
5. Sprouts will begin to appear within 24 hours (give or take, depending on what it is you are sprouting).
6. Make sure you rinse and drain the sprouts (as in soaking step 4 and sprouting steps 1–4) at least once or twice daily until they have reached the desired growth or are ready to be used.
7. Rinse your sprouts/nuts/grains/beans before eating.
8. They can be stored in the fridge in an airtight jar with a solid lid. Enjoy within 2 or 3 days.

## Quick Tips

Do not let buckwheat sprouts grow longer than the seed itself, to prevent unwanted quantities of the toxin fagopyrin, which can cause light sensitivity.

When choosing almonds, opt for unpasteurized. Due to a 2007 salmonella outbreak, California almonds are now pasteurized. California almonds are approximately 70 percent of the almonds eaten in the United States. Due to the pasteurization (heated to 160°F [71°C]) soaking will still activate the nut and help eliminate the phytic acid; however, they will not sprout.

Growing your own sprouts and microgreens is quite easy and fun. To learn how to get started, see our resources section on page 216.

### Please note

Sprouts can be subject to contamination that can result in bacterial growth such as *E. coli*, leading to food-borne illnesses. Always purchase fresh organic products from a reputable source, wash your hands thoroughly before handling foods and keep sprouting equipment and your kitchen clean to avoid any contamination. Make sure you consume them fresh out of the fridge and within three or four days (or cook them if desired).

## Hydration

Hydration is as important as any other part of your plant-powered diet because it affects everything else. Your health, performance, body composition, sleep, recovery, mental focus and even joint health are all dependent on proper hydration.

### Hydration and Performance

Muscles are composed of about 70 percent water and staying adequately hydrated can mean the difference between a great gym session and a mediocre one. Even mild dehydration can cause early fatigue, making your workout far more challenging than it should be.

During long-distance endurance sports, our muscles are craving more energy (oxygen) to sustain their effort. If your body is not sufficiently hydrated, it will reduce blood flow to your whole body, including your hard-working muscles. When the muscles do not get adequately supplied with blood, oxygen delivery will be reduced and, therefore, your performance will go down. Proper hydration before, during and after exercise will help keep your muscles primed and fueled to perform efficiently during a long workout or a race.

Water is essential for digestion, elimination, metabolization, hormonal balance and waste removal. Dehydration slows down all these chemical reactions, which can affect the rate at which you burn your calories for energy, which in the long term can then lead to excess body fat. Adequate water means proper digestion, an optimally running metabolism and the ability to burn calories at a higher rate. This not only helps keep your body fat levels in check but gives you more energy, helps with recovery and allows you to feel livelier throughout the day.

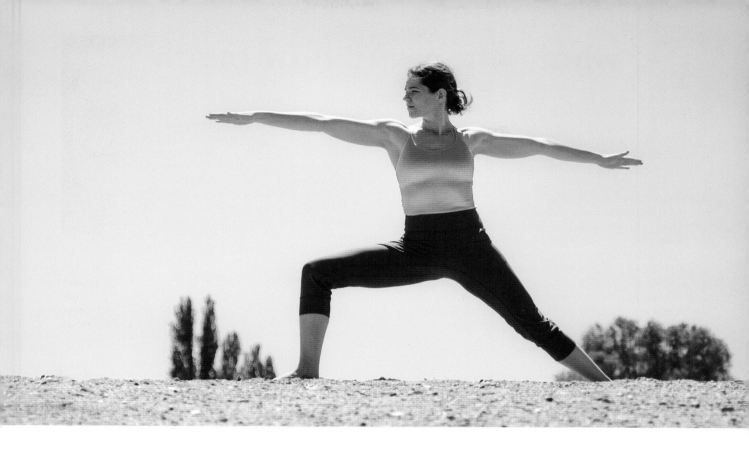

## Tips on Maintaining Hydration

You lose water every day through breathing, sweating and waste removal, so the need to replace the water lost through bodily functions is quite important.

- Do not wait until you are thirsty to drink water— by then, you are already quite dehydrated. Get in the habit of drinking water within 10 minutes of waking up, to replace the fluid that you lost during the night. This postsleep rehydration is especially important when performing a morning workout. Sometimes we like to mix it up and drink plain coconut water, or coconut water with a bit of lemon juice, to rehydrate and get ready for the day.

- Your body can effectively absorb only about a cup (240 ml) of fluid at once, so sip water throughout the day to help maintain hydration rather than gulping large amounts of $H_2O$ only a couple of times a day.

- One of the many benefits of the Plant-Powered Diet is that the food we eat is intensely hydrating. Therefore, it's not necessary to drink large amounts of fluids. Raw fruits and vegetables come packed with water. When food is cooked, especially at high temperatures, it loses the majority of its water content and, as a result, these foods can act as a sponge, pulling water from the body, increasing thirst. Furthermore, processed foods require more fluids to aid in digestion.

- Lastly, we recommend that you hydrate only with pure water. If you live in a city and depend on municipal water, it might be a good idea to invest in a water filtration system that will suit your needs. Ideally, you want to filter the water you use both for drinking and bathing, as immersing yourself in contaminated water may be even more hazardous to your health than drinking it.

# what, when and how much

## Nutrient Timing for Peak Performance

**If you love life, don't waste time,
for time is what life is made up of.
—Bruce Lee**

So far, we have covered the foundational principles of the Plant-Powered Diet. If you choose to apply them into your daily life, you will begin to notice significant improvements to your overall health in no time. That's our promise. Once this healthy foundation is firmly established, we can start to tailor our nutrition to support individual athletic goals. The timing of meals, combined with specially formulated recipes, is an effective strategy that could make a significant difference in your performance, body composition, energy levels, sleep quality and recovery after workouts.

Nutrient timing means eating specific nutrients, such as carbohydrates or protein, in a specific amount at specific times, such as before, during or after exercise, to promote health, athletic performance and to get or stay lean. This approach is based on how the body handles different nutrients at different times. Eating specific types of foods when your body is best able to use its nutrients is an incredibly powerful strategy that can help repair tissue damage, restore energy, replenish glycogen stores and promote muscle growth. On the other hand, if we fail to nourish our body properly before, during or after workout sessions, we are greatly diminishing our results from training. I am aware that this whole subject might sound complicated and perhaps a little nerdy. I used to be intimidated by the idea of "timing" my meals, but please trust me; it's not that hard. Read on and learn more about it, experiment with the recipes in this book and put the knowledge into practice. The results are 100 percent worth it!

There are three distinct phases of nutrient timing:

- Energy Phase (just before and during a workout)
- Anabolic Phase (up to 3 hours postworkout)
- Growth Phase (remainder of the day)

## Energy Phase
Just before and during a workout:

- We often get asked, "What is the best food to fuel my workout?" and while the preworkout snack and "during workout" fuel can be quite useful, making sure that you recover properly from your previous workout is far more critical. With that said, focus on supporting your body on an ongoing basis with nourishing foods rather than emphasizing an immediate preworkout fuel.

- The primary goal of fueling before and during training is to have enough energy to sustain your strength and endurance during the training session. Carbohydrates provide this energy, and you should always aim to enter your training sessions well fueled. However, because of differences in body composition, the ability to digest food and intensity of the sport, as well as individual goals (weight loss, muscle gain, etc.), one strategy may not work for all.

- Keep in mind that protein is for building muscle, not fueling up. If you emphasize protein instead of carbohydrates immediately before exercise, to burn as fuel, it will burn "dirty," meaning you will create a toxic environment in your body and hinder your workout performance.

- Being adequately hydrated before and during exercise will decrease the amount of stress placed on your body, allowing your body to work harder and perform better as well as speed up recovery time.

- A great goal to set for yourself is to never become thirsty or hungry during training!

The ratio of carbohydrates, fats and protein in the preworkout snack are determined by the intensity and duration of the activity. Keep in mind that every athlete's fuel requirements are slightly different, depending on their fitness level, the quality of their diet and to a lesser degree, genetic makeup.

| **LOW INTENSITY** | **MODERATE INTENSITY** | **HIGH INTENSITY** |
|---|---|---|

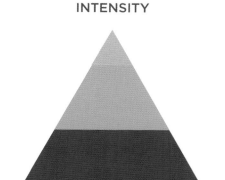

| 10% protein<br>70% fat<br>20% carbohydrates | 5% protein<br>35% fat<br>60% carbohydrates | 3% protein<br>7% fat<br>90% carbohydrates |
|---|---|---|

### Low-Intensity Activity (lasting more than three hours)

Biking, long-distance cycling, ultra marathon, triathlon, hiking, long walk, any job that requires sustained physical efforts.

#### Preworkout

Those training for an Ironman, ultra race or any activity lasting over three hours, the fitter and more trained you are, the higher percentage of fat is going to be used to fuel your performance. This fat-burning zone is a critical training zone for endurance athletes; it teaches the body to become efficient at using fat for fuel, saving glycogen (carbohydrate stored in the muscle), resulting in better endurance and eliminating the possibility of running out of energy and "hitting the wall." However, even a fraction of time spent in the fat-burning zone will burn muscle if not enough amino acids are present, therefore make sure also to include a small amount of protein. A good preworkout meal to support this level of exercise would be the Creamy Mango-Chia Pudding (page 87).

#### During

If your training session is longer than two hours, make sure to hydrate and replenish electrolytes as well as consume easily digestible nutrients, about every 25 minutes. Great options would be pure coconut water or our Salted Caramel Endurance Gel (page 118).

### Moderate-Intensity Activity (lasting anywhere between one and three hours)

Intense cycling, half marathon, Olympic distance triathlon, power hiking, dancing, skiing, canoeing, paddleboarding, doubles tennis.

#### Preworkout

To sustain moderate-intensity training, 40 percent of the energy must come from carbohydrates. If carbohydrate availability is compromised, fatigue will occur. One to two hours before your training session, also consume a small amount of easily digestible fat (ground chia or flax) and protein (hemp). A great option is the Coco-Mango Performance Bar (page 122).

#### During

Sip an electrolyte-rich drink every ten to fifteen minutes, or more often, during exercise, depending on such variables as heat and humidity as well as the intensity of your workout (basically the more you sweat, the more you want to replenish). Also, to sustain your performance, it may be very beneficial to consume easily digestible carbohydrates (agave or dates) during training sessions. A great choice that will cover both nutritional needs (electrolytes + carbohydrates) would be our Cucumber-Lime Chia Fresca (page 96).

## High-Intensity Activity (lasting anywhere between one and three hours)

Intense weight lifting workout, hard gym session, high-intensity interval training, 3 to 6 mile (5 to 10 km) run, any sport that involves quick, intense movements, such as tennis, soccer, hockey, basketball, squash/racquetball.

### Preworkout

The most efficient fuel to consume right before a high-intensity workout session is simple carbohydrates. Choose foods that will give you quick energy but won't take much time and effort to digest. Fresh fruit is the healthiest choice, and dates are also an excellent option. One of our go-to pregym snacks is a few Medjool dates with a touch of almond butter.

### During

If your workout is going to last more than 60 minutes, then you will need to replenish every 20 minutes after one hour of intense activity if you want to keep the body sufficiently fueled. A great way to sustain your energy and keep your stomach happy is Ginger Ale Workout Tonic (page 114).

## Anabolic Phase (0 to 45 minutes postexercise)

- If you are an athlete or train like one, then your workout isn't fully complete until you've refueled. The anabolic phase occurs within 45 minutes postexercise, during which time you will want to refuel with the proper nutrients so as to make gains in muscle mass, endurance and strength.

- Your postworkout snack should be very similar to your preworkout snack. Consume simple, easy-to-digest carbohydrates first, as they will help replenish lost glycogen (fuel for the cells) and provide your body with enough glucose to initiate the recovery process. Basically, if you don't replenish glycogen rapidly, your performance will suffer next time you train and you may even lose some muscle along the way.

- A protein-rich meal should be consumed later (45 to 90 minutes after your workout). The order is important for proper muscle building and strengthening to take place.

- Aim to consume a 3:1 to 4:1 ratio of carbs-to-protein, in a snack or beverage, as soon as you finish your workout. A great choice would be our Postrun Juice (page 100) or Pineapple + Spirulina in a Jar (page 178).

## Growth Phase (45 minutes postworkout to the beginning of the next workout)

There are two parts of the growth phase:

### 45 to 90 Minutes Postworkout

- Forty-five to 90 minutes after a workout is an ideal time for a complete, nutrient-rich meal consisting of 10 to 20 grams of high-quality, easily digestible raw protein (such as hemp hearts or chia), omega-3 fatty acids (hemp hearts and flaxseeds) and vitamins and minerals from natural food sources.

- If your training session was extra intense, a liquid meal is the best option. A Raw Power Smoothie (page 104) is our go-to postworkout choice as it's quick to make, easy to digest and assimilate and contains all the necessary nutrients for health, growth and repair.

- If you have a postworkout substantial (solid) meal, include dark leafy greens for added vitamin and antioxidant support and clean plant-based protein, such as quinoa, buckwheat, beans, lentils, algae, nuts and seeds. A great choice at this time would be the Pesto Quinoa Bowl (page 150).

### In between Workouts (3 to 22 hours)

For optimal health and performance, eat clean, whole, alkaline-forming, nutrient-rich, plant-based foods daily, as described in detail in the previous sections. Eating this way will help replenish the nutrients lost during your training sessions and promote optimal health.

The secret to fatigue-proofing your body and speeding recovery from your workouts comes down to consuming alkaline-forming foods. When you exercise, you essentially tear your muscles and produce a lot of acid, in the form of lactic acid. That's why you get sore, yet that's also the initial stimulus that helps your muscles grow. Replenishing with whole plant-based foods will speed up the healing process and reduce inflammation in the body.

By following the Plant-Powered Diet, you'll find you recover faster from your workouts, minimize illness and injury, and you'll have far more energy because your blood is healthy and able to properly transport energy-giving oxygen throughout your body.

## Natural Weight Loss

All too often, when people hear about the Plant-Based Diet, it sparks a question: Will it help me lose weight? Let me approach this question first by acknowledging that only a healthy body can achieve normal weight.

It never ceases to amaze me how many weight-loss programs promise quick-fix solutions to shed pounds and "proven tips" to lose weight. Unfortunately, many so-called weight-loss experts fail to acknowledge that losing weight and achieving a healthy lean body is about healing. Our body is an amazing machine, and it never behaves irrationally. If it gets overloaded with stress, environmental toxins, nutritional deficiencies, too many calories, too little sleep and many, many more imbalances, it will not be able to digest and metabolize food efficiently. This chronic physical and emotional stress will result in toxicity and excess body weight.

Common factors that cause weight gain:

- Eating a highly processed diet of nutrient-depleted foods
- Overconsumption of acid-forming foods and supplements
- Overworking
- Overtraining
- Overstimulation of senses
- Exhaustion
- Lack of sleep
- Irregular eating habits
- Heavy meals at nighttime
- Overeating
- Stimulants such as coffee, tea and cigarettes
- Not drinking enough water
- Feeling unfulfilled and dissatisfied
- Alcohol consumption
- Unresolved conflicts (impairing digestion)
- Fear, worry and other emotional upsets
- Environmental toxins and pollution (air, water, soil)

If your goal is to lose body fat and achieve a healthy weight, forget the newest crash diet, extreme workouts, supplements or diet pills and put your attention on reducing stress, detoxifying and healing your body. Consider the following strategies to help you reach your goals.

## Healthy Weight Loss Strategies

- Eat primarily organic plant-based foods that are minimally-processed.
- Eat smaller meals throughout the day.
- Favor alkaline-forming, low-calorie, nutrient-rich raw foods.
- Slow down your meals and enjoy each bite of your food.
- Do not eat when ill or upset.
- Hydrate with pure water.
- Prioritize a good night's sleep.
- Maintain emotional balance. Release worry, fear and anxiety, jealousy, stress and resentment through physical exercise and deep breathing.
- Live in a place that contributes to good health (fresh, clean air, low crime rate, etc.).
- Develop loving and supportive relationships with your partner, family and friends.

Your health and body composition will improve automatically once you remove toxicity and keep your body and mind open and clean. If weight loss is your goal, you might greatly benefit from our 24-Week Guided Program—The Plant-Based Solution; see the details in the resources section on page 216.

## Lean Muscle Building

The best way to build new muscle tissue is to regularly challenge your body with intense resistance training and nourish it with the right building blocks.

When it comes to training, choose exercises that are difficult yet safe and that you enjoy. Make strength training part of your lifestyle. Each time you train, you will create small microtears in your muscles as you challenge your body with more repetitions and heavier weights. This micro breakdown in the muscle tissue doesn't stop at the end of the workout; it continues even after your last rep. That's why proper nourishment is a crucial component of muscle growth. By giving your body the right nutrients it needs to repair these tears, your muscles will rebuild, growing bigger and stronger. Following the principles of the Plant-Powered Diet is an ideal place to start; however, if your goal is to build lean muscle mass, you will have to put particular emphasis on the amount of food you consume—you'll need plenty of lean protein, quality carbs and healthy fats, too.

## Lean Protein

Protein is the building block of muscle tissue, and you will need quality protein, in larger quantities than nonathletes, to grow and maintain lean muscle. Protein comprises a variety of amino acids; some amino acids are essential to obtain from the diet; others, your body can produce itself. By including a variety of lean, plant-based protein sources, you ensure that your amino acid needs are being met. How much protein do you need to gain lean muscle? Over the years, I have found that most people, myself included, who eat a whole food plant-based diet and lift weights regularly need roughly 0.5 to 0.75 grams of protein per pound (455 g) of bodyweight each day to achieve their desired body composition. So, if your goal is to be 130 pounds (59 kg), lean, muscular and vibrant, then you will want to aim for a minimum of 75 grams of high-quality, bio-available plant-based protein per day.

## Quality Carbohydrates

Although some diet approaches give carbs a bad rap, when you're building muscle, carbs are just as important as protein. Carbohydrates provide your body with energy. Muscles can store energy from carbohydrates (in the form of glycogen) and use them as fuel during workouts. However, because muscles can only store a limited amount of these carbs, you have to consume more before, during and after your training session. By doing this, it will give you the energy you need to fuel a powerful workout and allow you to recover faster.

## Healthy Fats

Don't neglect fat in your diet, even if your goal is to shed body fat while you build or maintain lean muscle. Healthy fats, such as cold-pressed oils, nuts, seeds, avocado, chia and hemp, play an important role in metabolizing the food you eat. Without dietary fat, your body cannot absorb vitamins A, D, E and K. Fat is also essential in the production of hormones, necessary for the lubrication of joints and helps protect muscle tissue from breaking down.

Overall, if your goal is to gain lean muscle, you need to step outside your comfort zone regularly. Train hard, eat clean, keep your thoughts positive and you will see results! We offer a Six-Week Lean & Strong Program to get you started; see the resources section on page 216 for more details.

## Cravings

Food cravings are powerful signals from our brains, letting us know that we are not eating a well-balanced diet or that our body may be missing out on a variety of vitamins and minerals. Monitoring and understanding these cravings will help you fine-tune your nutrition to further improve your overall health and athletic performance.

### How to Put Cravings in Their Place

Following the principles of the Plant-Powered Diet will provide your body with complete nourishment, so you will feel satisfied and have less room for processed and nutrient-depleted food. You can satisfy your cravings easily by choosing healthier alternatives that supply you with the key nutrients your body is craving.

### Craving chocolate?

This can be a deficiency of magnesium, B vitamins, chromium and/or essential fatty acids.

**Troubleshoot it with:** dark leafy greens, pumpkin seeds, lentils or avocado, or treat yourself to a Chocolate Muscle Mylk (page 112).

### Craving salty foods?

It could be an indication you have a mineral imbalance and that you actually are lacking in sodium. Also, that you are not hydrating enough!

**Troubleshoot it with:** sea vegetables, such as nori, kelp or dulse. Enjoy some coconut water or fresh celery juice. Stay away from table salt, which is stripped of its minerals; instead, sprinkle Celtic sea salt or Himalayan pink salt at every meal. And hydrate with pure water.

### Craving bread?

It could mean you are not getting enough amino acids.

Amino acids are the building blocks of protein. One amino acid in particular, tryptophan, is needed to synthesize the mood-regulating brain chemical serotonin, which can be lacking in the diet.

**Troubleshoot it by:** upping your protein, consuming hemp, chia, quinoa, nuts and tryptophan-containing foods, such as buckwheat, cacao, cashews, walnuts and bananas.

### Craving sugar?

Sweet cravings are caused by low energy or fatigue, as well as dehydration. It's a survival signal for quick energy. When your blood sugar is low, your brain signals an urgent need for sugar. When your muscles are glycogen-depleted, you experience a craving for carbs until your muscles are adequately replenished.

**Troubleshoot it with:** fruits, such as apples, pears and berries, and starchy carbohydrates, such as sweet potatoes, squash, plantains, pseudograins and legumes.

### Craving pizza, cheese and fried foods?

Cravings for food high in fat could indicate you're not getting enough healthy fats throughout the day. Don't shy away from fat! It helps fuel your brain, keeps you sharp and focused and improves your mood! It's also needed to boost immunity and send signals to the glands to produce hormones. Also, consumption of fat during a meal helps you feel full since it's slow to digest. Another bonus? Eating fat actually helps you lose excess fat from your body!

**Troubleshoot it with:** avocados, sun-dried olives, almond butter, walnuts, seeds and coconut yogurt.

### Craving coffee or a midafternoon/midmorning pick-me-up?

Your body is looking for energy! Besides the fact that coffee contains an addictive chemical (caffeine), take notice that maybe you are craving the sugar that you put into it. Regardless of whether you are craving a pick-me up treat, your body is looking for energy. But since coffee is a stimulant, it ends up depleting some of your body's mineral stores, causing you to end up feeling worn out later on in the day.

**Troubleshoot it by:** choosing the enzyme-rich Raw Power Smoothie (page 104), green tea, Matcha Latte (page 80) or fresh green juice instead.

### Emotional Factors

Cravings don't necessarily always stem from an inadequate amount of nutrients. Sadness, boredom, stress, lack of fulfillment, poor self-esteem, negative body image (and the list goes on) may trigger the desire to fill a void using food. I personally struggled with emotional eating for many years, and food was my "drug" of choice that temporarily distracted me from uncomfortable feelings. This "distraction" created a very unhealthy and deeply rooted cycle that was not easy to break. If emotional eating is holding you back from having the body you want and most important, from the well-being you deserve, then read on. In the following pages, I will share several lifestyle habits that have been profoundly helpful along my journey to vibrant health, and perhaps you, too, might discover the missing piece for your life's puzzle.

## What about Supplements?

As someone who cares about athletic performance and results from training, you may consider supplementing your diet with protein powders, vitamins, minerals or other products that claim to help you get lean, grow big muscles and turn you into an overnight superhero. However, before you go ahead and invest in any commercial supplements, understand that many are inefficient or ineffective, while others are downright dangerous. When you examine the ingredients on the label of the majority of these products, you will find a bunch of acid-forming synthetic ingredients, such as food coloring, artificial sweeteners, refined carbohydrates, highly processed proteins and sometimes even harmful fats. From personal experience, we have found that the most efficient way to achieve your fitness goals is through practical training combined with optimal nutrition. Rather than trusting cheaply made, poor-quality supplements, feed your body with plenty of natural, clean, toxin-free, nutrient-rich plant foods and supplement with superfoods instead.

### Superfoods for Peak Performance

Complementing the Plant-Powered Diet with supplements in the form of whole superfoods can offer additional advantages to your overall health and performance. The following is a list of foods we have used over the years to help build muscular, lean, healthy bodies. Some of these foods can be found at your local grocery store, while others you can source online. Check the resources section on page 216 for details.

### Greens

As we previously mentioned, green leafy vegetables are some of the most health-promoting foods to include in our Plant-Powered Diet. Why count them as superfoods? Nutritionally, they are an excellent source of calcium, and they are vitamin and mineral rich. They're also alkaline-forming and full of active enzymes. They are affordable and accessible and you can choose from a large variety to find the ones that you enjoy; lettuce greens, kale, spinach, arugula, mustard greens, endive, parsley, cilantro . . .

**Nutritional superpowers:** alkaline-forming, vitamins, calcium, iron, strength and muscle building

### Celery

Celery is an absolute staple of a plant-powered diet. It's high in natural sodium, making it a great choice for those looking to build muscle and strength. It's also high in water, perfect for a postworkout juice to help replenish valuable fluids lost during exercise. It contains apigenin—a substance known for reducing inflammation.

**Nutritional superpowers:** anti-inflammatory, rich in fiber, adrenal support

### Sea Vegetables

Nori, dulse, kelp and other sea vegetables are a powerhouse of nutrition. They are loaded with minerals and trace elements that provide a convenient way to increase natural mineral content in our diet, including healthful sodium and iron. Add a pinch of kelp flakes to your water to replenish electrolytes lost during a workout. Incorporate dried seaweed into your dressings and soups or use nori sheets to make raw Veggie Nori Rolls (page 143).

**Nutritional superpowers:** alkaline-forming, calcium, electrolytes, iron, iodine

### Fresh Young Coconut

We buy young coconuts, which you can find in most Asian food markets. Prices can range from $1.50 to $5.00 (USD) per coconut, depending on where you get them. We crack it open and pour the water into a jar. Coconut water, especially when sourced from fresh whole coconuts, is one of the most potent forms of natural electrolytes. Although many athletes turn to sports drinks that are full of processed sugars, artificial flavors and additives, coconut water is a natural alternative to keep hydrated. After straining the water out of the nut, we scoop out the "meat" or "flesh" and use it for yogurts, smoothies or dressings. This jellylike substance on the inside of the coconut helps restore oxidative tissue damage and contains a source of healthy fats, proteins and various vitamins and minerals.

**Nutritional superpowers:** Muscle building, rich in fiber, iron, amino acids

### Bananas

We love bananas. Personally, I believe that they are one of the best foods an athlete can consume during training and throughout the rest of the day. They are cheap, superversatile, portable and the healthiest option in a convenience store. Bananas are a great source of potassium, so they're ideal after a hard, sweaty session and also can help keep your muscles from cramping. On days when you are falling behind on calories, eat a few bananas to get you back on track.

**Nutritional superpowers:** source of energy, potassium, iron, vitamin C

### Pseudograins

Pseudograins are not exactly grains; they are seeds, but make an excellent substitute for common grains. Buckwheat, quinoa, amaranth, millet and wild rice are all gluten-free, easily digestible and suitable for those who have celiac disease or are sensitive to gluten. The nutritional value of pseudograins is far superior to that of most other foods. All of them are alkaline-forming and add a substantial amount of protein to your plant-powered diet, especially when they are sprouted.

**Nutritional superpowers:** protein rich, B vitamins, calcium, iron

### Dates

Dates are a beneficial fruit to fuel your workouts because they provide clean-burning energy, not to mention they are delicious. The high-glycemic carb content in dates allows the liver to convert this glucose into glycogen, the primary source of energy for an endurance athlete. Therefore, dates serve as fuel before, during and after your athletic training.

**Nutritional superpowers:** energy for endurance, iron, potassium, fiber

## Goji Berries

These little delicious red berries are a real nutrition powerhouse. Nutritionally, they are an incredible source of protein and antioxidants, containing 18 amino acids, including all 9 essential amino acids and over 20 vitamins and minerals, such as vitamin C, zinc, riboflavin (vitamin $B_2$), calcium and iron. Incorporate them in your salads, smoothies and snacks to help combat inflammation and promote muscle growth. Always seek raw, sun-dried, certified organic goji berries.

**Nutritional superpowers:** protein rich, vitamin C, antioxidants, calcium, iron

## Camu Camu Berries

Camu camu is an Amazon rainforest fruit that contains 60 times more vitamin C than an orange. It also packs a potent blend of amino acids, such as serine, leucine and valine, which play crucial roles in muscle and bone tissue growth and recovery. Fresh camu camu is not easy to find and is hard on the taste buds—it's very sour. Go with a powder; you can mix about a teaspoon into recovery drinks, smoothies and juices for a plant-powered boost, especially during cold and flu season.

**Nutritional superpowers:** boosts immune system, vitamin C, antioxidants, anti-inflammatory

## Hemp

Hemp is packed with over twenty amino acids, including the nine essential amino acids your body must acquire through diet. It's also rich in essential fatty acids that support the function of the cardiovascular, immune and nervous systems, as well as help reduce inflammation in the body—all of which are important for long-term athletic performance. Sprinkle hemp hearts on your salad or smoothie bowl, or add to dressings, soups or energy bars. Hemp protein is made from hemp seeds, doesn't require any heat processing and is considered one of the cleanest proteins available. Add a tablespoon (8 g) of natural organic, raw and unprocessed hemp protein to smoothies or juices.

**Nutritional superpowers:** complete protein, fiber, calcium, iron, omega-6 and omega-3

## Flaxseeds

Flax is a vital addition to a plant-based diet, especially for athletes. High in omega-3 fatty acids, flaxseeds help reduce inflammation caused by exercise as well as encourage the body to burn fat as fuel. To get the most out of flax, in terms of omega-3s, fiber and other nutrients, grind the seeds before you eat them. Add them to your smoothie, sprinkle on salads or incorporate them into your power bars.

**Nutritional superpowers:** omega-3s, anti-inflammatory, burns fat, fiber

## Chia Seeds

Because of its omega profile, chia seeds get compared to flaxseeds. Both are rich in omega-3, but chia can be eaten whole and doesn't need to ground like flax to make it digestible. Aztec warriors were rumored to eat chia before going into battle, to boost their energy and endurance. They were also said to have carried it with them when they ran long distances, to use as their body's primary fuel source. These little seeds come packed with trace minerals, vitamins and essential fats and are an excellent source of complete plant protein.

**Nutritional superpowers:** complete protein, omega-3s, fiber, boosts endurance

## Spirulina

Spirulina is a type of algae, and it also happens to be one of the oldest life forms on Earth. It is a high-energy, nutrient-rich food that helps nourish, detoxify and alkalize the body. Spirulina has more protein than meat, fish, poultry and soybeans. It contains the most beta-carotene of any food as well as all the essential amino acids and no fewer than ten nonessential ones. It is also rich in iron, vitamins A, E and B, potassium, enzymes, minerals and phytonutrients—major disease-fighters. Include spirulina powder into your postworkout drinks, smoothies or juices, or take spirulina tablets with water.

**Nutritional superpowers:** complete protein, boosts energy, iron, B vitamins

## Chlorella

These microscopic plants that grow in freshwater offer high levels of digestible, alkaline-forming protein. Chlorella is also known for having the highest chlorophyll content of all plants. Chlorophyll—a pigment that gives plants their green color—is prized for its ability to cleanse our blood by helping remove toxins deposited from dietary and environmental sources. Chlorophyll is also linked to the body's production of red blood cells, therefore improving energy levels and contributing to peak athletic performance. If you choose to take a chlorella supplement, look for one with cracked cell walls so your body can easily digest its goodness. Add it to your smoothies or juices, or mix a teaspoon or two into your water.

**Nutritional superpowers:** high protein, vitamin D, cleansing and detoxifying

## Turmeric

One of India's most treasured spices, turmeric contains curcumin—an anti-inflammatory powerhouse. It helps reduce muscle and joint pain and improve recovery from exercise, which leads to more consistent training and higher intensity levels, leading to increased performance. You can add either dried turmeric or grated fresh to your meals or smoothies. To activate the antioxidant curcumin, add a pinch of black pepper.

**Nutritional superpowers:** recovery, anti-inflammatory, pain reliever

## Maca

The native population has consumed this Peruvian root vegetable for centuries. The Incas claimed it cured a long list of disorders, including depression, infertility, low libido, bone weakness, anemia and chronic fatigue. Inca warriors even consumed it as a prebattle energy boost. In the Western world, maca is prized for its nutrient density, positive effects on energy and potential to support the endocrine system. Add a teaspoon of maca powder to your postworkout smoothie—this will help with recovery and normalize stress levels.

**Nutritional superpowers:** increase energy and stamina, rich in amino acids, hormone balance

## Vitamin B$_{12}$

There is a common question we get asked: whether vegetarians, vegans and plant-based eaters can get enough vitamin B$_{12}$. The answer is quite important because a deficiency in B$_{12}$ is pretty serious and today 40 to 60 percent of the population in North America is B$_{12}$ deficient, including those on a meat-eating diet. Vitamin B$_{12}$ (also known as cobalamin) is essential to our health. It plays a vital role in the normal functioning of the brain and nervous system and the formation of red blood cells. It also helps regulate and synthesize DNA as well as the brain chemicals serotonin and dopamine, critical "feel good" hormones.

Common side effects of B$_{12}$ deficiency include:

- Fatigue/tiredness
- Muscle weakness
- Constipation or diarrhea
- Loss of appetite/weight loss
- Anemia
- Stress/inability to handle stress
- Menstrual/fertility problems
- Tingling or numbness in the hands or feet
- Mental/memory problems
- Vision loss

What you might not know is that this vitamin is produced by bacteria found in soil as well as in the guts of animals (including humans)—but for the bacteria to make B$_{12}$, the soil needs to contain the mineral cobalt. Believe it or not, historically most of us would receive a sufficient amount of B$_{12}$ daily by merely being in close contact with farm animals, since the feces of cow, chicken, sheep and many other animals all contain large amounts of active B$_{12}$. When these feces were regularly used as manure to grow crops, B$_{12}$ was consumed as a residue bacteria living on unsanitized vegetables. And here is where the problem lies: Due to declining soil quality from intensive overfarming, making the soil deficient in cobalt, and because our vegetables are superwashed, vegans, vegetarians and other plant-based eaters don't get enough B$_{12}$ without supplementation and fortification. However, B$_{12}$ deficiency isn't just a problem for plant-based eaters. Absorption of B$_{12}$ requires a healthy gut. Problems with any part of the digestive system make a vitamin B$_{12}$ deficiency possible. For anyone who does not want to risk the 60 percent chance of becoming deficient and wants to enjoy a healthy and happy life, oral supplementation is the simplest way to avoid a B$_{12}$ deficiency.

## Restore

It would be ideal for getting all the minerals we need from food. Our goal is to one day grow our organic food in a highly mineralized soil away from pollution and chemicals. However, until then, we have decided to support our health with a mineral supplement. Restore is a fantastic product, and you only need a tiny amount each day to keep your body and mind functioning at peak performance. You can find more information in the resources section on page 216.

**Nutritional superpowers:** mental clarity, better sleep, gut health

Please note that you should discuss any new supplements or foods with your health-care provider. People taking certain medications should also be careful when using any herbs or superfoods or supplementing with them.

# rest, relax and restore

## Sleep, Meditation and Breath

*Your health is what you make of it. Everything you do and think either adds to the vitality, energy and spirit you possess or takes away from it.*
-Ann Wigmore

I am a firm believer that nutrient-dense food and intense exercise is a must for improved fitness and good health. However, the quality of our life and health depends on a lot more than just the food we eat and the way we train.

Success at anything starts with the ability to cope with stress effectively. If you want to enjoy optimal health, it is important to learn to manage your stress level—or it will ultimately negatively affect you and your performance. What I'm about to share with you in this chapter are everyday practices to help you relieve stress, clear your mind, get more out of your workouts, speed recovery and give you lasting energy so that you can make each day amazing.

### Sleep

Proper sleep is essential for elite performance and healthy life. Up to 90 percent of muscle growth occurs during deep sleep. Getting a good night's sleep will not only help your body repair and recover, but is also crucial for your emotional health, keeping you happy and mentally focused. On the other hand, recurring nights of lousy sleep will pile on body fat, mess with your hormones, make you more susceptible to chronic illnesses, steal your energy and drain your spirit.

Sleep can be divided into two main parts—before midnight and after midnight. For adults, the most critical processes of cleansing and repair occur during the two hours of sleep before midnight. This period involves deep sleep, often referred to as deep delta phase sleep. It lasts for about an hour from eleven p.m. to midnight. During this phase, you enter a dreamless state of sleep where oxygen consumption in the body drops—resulting in profound physical relaxation. Growth factors, commonly known as growth hormones, are released in abundance during this hour of deep sleep. These powerful hormones are responsible for cellular growth, repair and rejuvenation—people who don't produce enough growth hormones age faster. For the past few years, there has been a trend in the health and fitness world to consume synthetic growth hormones, which create "phenomenal" antiaging results, but can also have devastating side effects, including heart disease and cancer. On the other hand, if the body makes them, at the right time and in the correct amounts, as happens during deep delta sleep, they can keep the body vital and youthful at every age.

Deep sleep never occurs after midnight, and it comes only if you go to sleep at least two hours before midnight. If your stress levels are too high, your body will also not be able to get into a deep phase of sleep. If you miss out on deep sleep regularly, your body and mind become overtired. Not getting deep sleep triggers abnormal stress responses in the form of constant secretions of stress hormones, such as adrenaline, cortisol or cholesterol. To keep these artificially derived energy bursts going, at least for a while, you may be tempted to reach for stimulants, such as coffee, tea, candy, soda and alcohol. These stimulants will only feed a vicious cycle that will eventually lead to chronic fatigue. So, how do you fix a broken sleep pattern? You can naturally reduce your stress hormone levels, through clean plant-based nutrition, and supplementing with such ingredients as ashwagandha and maca (try the Sleep Tonic on page 115). Yoga, meditation and breathwork are also beneficial in reducing stress, as well as the simple act of doing more of what makes you happy.

### Meditation and Breath

All wellness starts in the mind. If the mind is well, the body can do amazing things. However, most of us lead a life that overloads the brain and makes us susceptible to stress. When we have nonstop demands and pressures of juggling work, home, health and personal responsibilities, this forces our nervous system to work overtime. It creates stress on our body and eventually leads to physical and mental imbalance. The greatest gift you can offer yourself is daily meditation. By creating the time to sit and breathe, you allow a gentle release of the pressure accumulated in your mind. Meditation will enable you to bring your body to a natural state of your well-being so you can flow through your day feeling balanced, calm and aligned.

Just sitting quietly and breathing, not to make something happen, but for the pleasure and comfort of your well-being is the foundation for meditation. It requires no intellect, only your pure awareness. Merely by breathing naturally, keeping the breath in mind, not attempting to control or force it—just mindfully noticing the in and out process of the breathing. When you can become aware of your breath and appreciate it, you will allow yourself to tune in to the present moment. Also, by aligning with the present, you invite silence and stillness—the essence of meditation. When you take the time to meditate, you promote inner balance and your health and well-being will be easy to maintain.

Relaxing and allowing is something I have had to make a conscious effort to do. My days, like those of most people, are jam-packed; setting aside fifteen minutes to slow down and switch off felt almost impossible. I used to do everything on my to-do list first, and if there was time left over, I would meditate. Then, one day, I finally decided to make meditation a priority. Although my life is still busy and at times a bit chaotic, meditation allows me to flow through my days more easily and effortlessly. I get sick less often and have tons more energy and stamina during my training sessions. I can focus better, keep my thoughts positive and resist distractions that pull me away from living a healthy, happy life filled with love and joy.

Meditation (like anything you wish to do well) requires practice and consistency. Personally, I use my breath to guide me, but you don't have to. Just allow yourself fifteen minutes a day to sit quietly, disconnect from this world and reconnect with the inner part of yourself.

If you are interested in meditation but struggle with how to begin or cultivate a consistent practice, see our resources section on page 216.

## Healthy Gut

**All disease begins in the gut.**
**-Hippocrates**

How well the body digests food, absorbs nutrients and eliminates waste has a direct influence on our overall well-being. A healthy gut, therefore, is not only an essential component of excellent health, but also plays a critical role in moving athletic performance to the next level. Taking good care of your digestive system can significantly influence how well you perform and how fast you recover and also impact your mental state, concentration and energy levels.

Digestion is the initial process through which our body receives nutrients from the food we eat. If your digestive tract, a.k.a. your gut, is out of balance, it can quickly destroy your overall nutrition. In other words, you could be eating the highest-quality, organic, nutrient-dense foods, but an unhealthy gut could deprive your whole body of important nutrients, so that the excellent nutrition from food goes to waste. Further along, this poorly digested waste must be removed from the body, and for that, we are equipped with a very efficient sewage system—the colon. However, the colon's ability to effectively eliminate waste is also dependent on a clean and healthy condition. A poorly functioning digestive system paired up with an overloaded colon is an absolute health hazard.

The following are some of the symptoms manifesting as a result of gut and colon imbalance:

- Digestive issues (gas, bloating)
- Constipation or diarrhea
- Food allergies or sensitivities
- Vitamin $B_{12}$ deficiency
- Candida
- Anxiety
- Depression
- Fatigue
- Mood swings, irritability
- Skin problems, such as eczema or rosacea
- Diabetes
- Autoimmune disease (leaky gut syndrome, IBS, Crohn's disease)
- Frequent infections (colds and flu)
- Poor memory and brain fog (difficulty concentrating)
- Neck and shoulder pain
- Lower back pain

### Ways to Improve Your Gut Health

One of the first things you can do to take care of your delicate gut is to feed it high-quality, nutrient-rich foods. Also, trust me, on the Plant-Powered Diet, there are so many wonderful ways to achieve this every single day. Green equals clean, so make sure to eat a big green salad each day: Packed with chlorophyll, enzymes and fiber, a leafy green salad is a powerhouse when it comes to good-for-your-gut foods.

Another great way to develop healthy gut flora is through probiotics. The word probiotic means "for life" or "promoting life." Probiotics hold the key not just for better health, a stronger immune system or helping heal digestive issues; they are also great at detoxing the body by controlling the bad bacteria in our gut. Fermented foods, such as sauerkraut (page 67), raw cultured veggies, kombucha, water-based kefir, coconut yogurt (page 55) and cultured plant-based cheeses (page 203) are all rich sources of probiotics; consume these regularly. You could also supplement with plant-based probiotics two or three times a week to keep the levels up. Look for broad-spectrum probiotic blends that have at least two strains (more is better) plus 1 billion organisms per serving in capsule or powdered form. It's important to note that many probiotic supplements do not actually survive in an unhealthy gut that is highly acidic; however, once a healthy environment is established—where probiotics can thrive (by eating more alkaline, raw and fermented foods)—the likelihood that microorganisms in probiotic supplements will provide benefits to the body goes up.

The next advice I would like to offer you is slowing down to eat and taking the time to chew your food well. Digestion actually begins in the mouth. The act of chewing food mixes it with our saliva; rich in digestive enzymes, saliva begins to break down the food even before it reaches our stomach. Therefore, the first step in improving your digestive problems is to chew your food thoroughly—the more your food is chewed up, the higher the absorption by your body.

Finally, let's talk about poop. Your bowel movement can reveal a lot about your gut, particularly the health of your colon. It is vital to have at least one bowel movement a day. If you wake up feeling groggy, heavy, dull, unmotivated and negative, the chances are that waste matter in your colon is backed up. This backup is quite an unhealthy situation as bowels that do not move frequently enough begin to accumulate toxins and poisons and are subject to harmful parasites, bacteria, mold and yeast. The standard American diet, specifically dairy products and white flour, act like glue in our intestines and eventually form a rubberlike layer, called mucoid plaque or biofilm, all through the bowels. This plaque causes inflammation, malabsorption, constipation or diarrhea, ulcers and perhaps even cancer. Sometimes the journey to vibrant health takes us to unusual places, and for me, colon hydrotherapy was one of them. From my experience, colon hydrotherapy, also called colon irrigation or colonic, is the most effective and safe way to cleanse the colon and restore the proper functioning of the intestinal tract. Within a 50- to 60-minute session, a colonic can eliminate large amounts of trapped waste that may have taken many years to accumulate. It may not be for everyone, so do your research, consult your health-care practitioner and decide for yourself whether this is the right approach for you. Either way, keep your bowels moving!

## Fasting

There's an ever-growing group of people, some elite athletes even, convinced that fasting could improve your health and help you lose fat. Is it true? Alternatively, just another fad? Is it healthy to not eat for most of the day, or even for several days in a row? How can your body properly function with no food? In this section, we will explore this subject and how it relates to the plant-powered lifestyle.

Fasting, in various forms, has been practiced for centuries as a method of healing the body, mind and spirit. In this day and age, it could be a very beneficial practice. However, it needs to be approached intelligently and not taken to the extreme. During a fast, we don't eat any food but drink plenty of pure water or fresh juice (preferably fruit juice). By eliminating food, we allow the body to do two things—rest and restore. Fasting gives the digestive system (pancreas, stomach, liver, intestines) and even the kidneys somewhat of a break, which provides the body with more energy to clean itself of toxic waste, and therefore promote healing.

Most of us fast, if only for just a few hours, every night. It's a great practice to consume your last meal of the day no later than two to three hours before bedtime. This time gives your body a chance to digest the food and allows for a deeper state of rest. Some people extend their evening fast by not eating until noon each day, or by allowing a longer period between their last meal and going to bed. This way of eating is often referred to as intermittent eating or intermittent fasting. Although these shorter-duration fasts tend to be more common, extended fasts could lead to deep healing and regeneration. Many people who try it become passionate advocates because the benefits can indeed be profound.

### Can Fasting Improve Athletic Performance?

Fasting can be one of the critical keys to unleashing new levels of athletic performance, enhancing recovery and promoting overall body regeneration. Fasting is, however, a short-term fix, a remedy, and will not make up for unhealthy habits and poor lifestyle choices. People who fast in hopes of improving performance, yet shortly after return to eating their typical diet consisting of processed foods, meats, dairy products and so forth, are merely wasting their time and stressing their system. The only key to optimum health and performance is consistency and dedication to efficient and effective training, combined with clean lifestyle choices, including eating a nutrient-rich diet.

### Where to Begin?

A good guideline is to start by going for twelve hours overnight without food and beverages other than pure water. For example, you would eat your last meal at seven p.m. and fast until seven a.m. the following morning. After you are used to twelve hours, you may want to experiment with a longer fasting time. Giving your body a rest from food, work and training one day a week can yield amazing results. However, if you are beginning your plant-based journey, my advice is to not worry about fasting yet. Educate yourself first, eliminate the intake of unhealthy food and progress from there.

In conclusion, fasting is not a shortcut to health, not a magic formula for a lean body, but another area that requires honesty and attention.

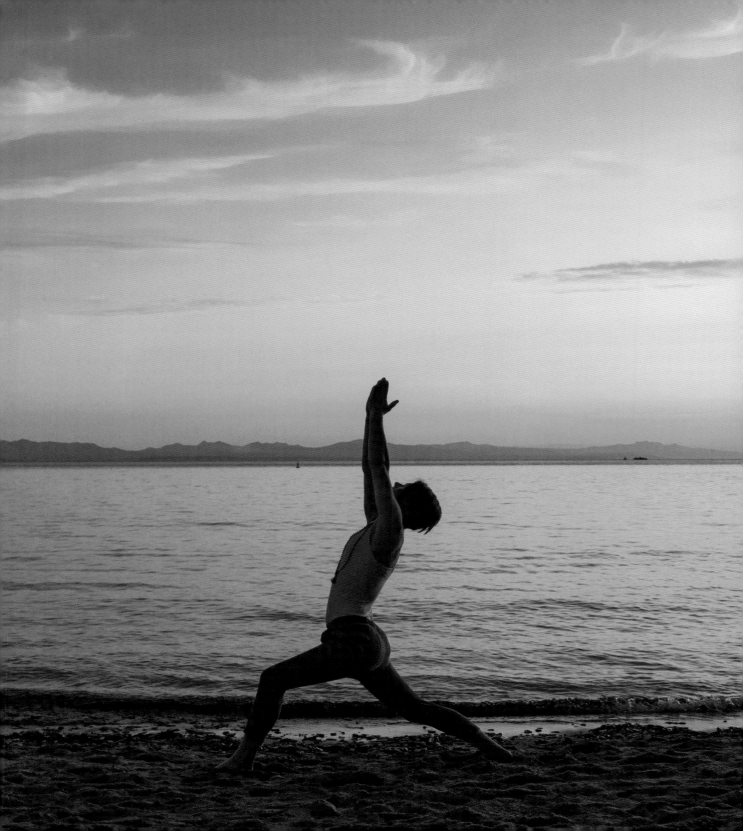

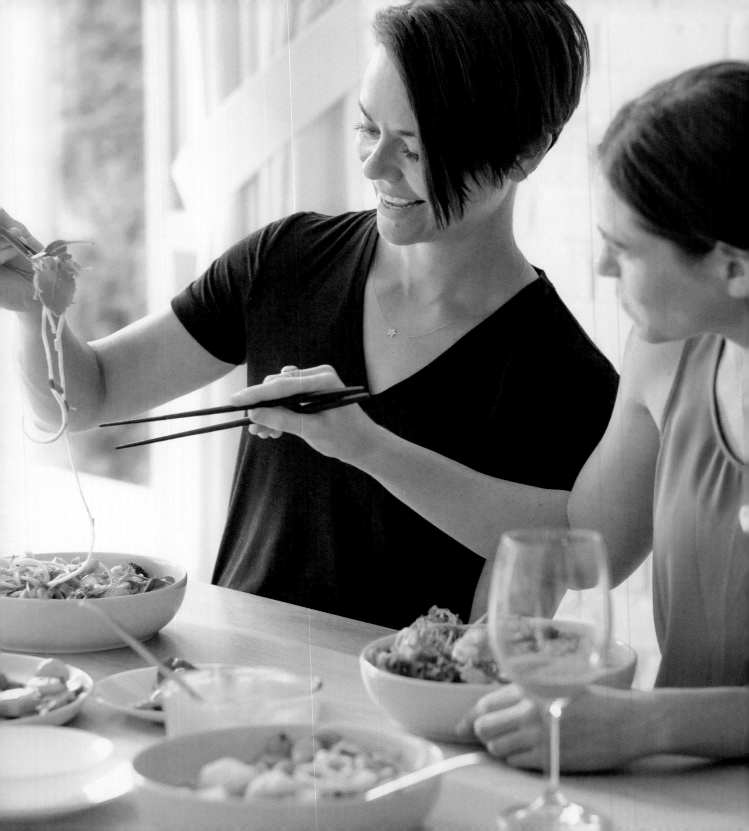

# plant-powered recipes

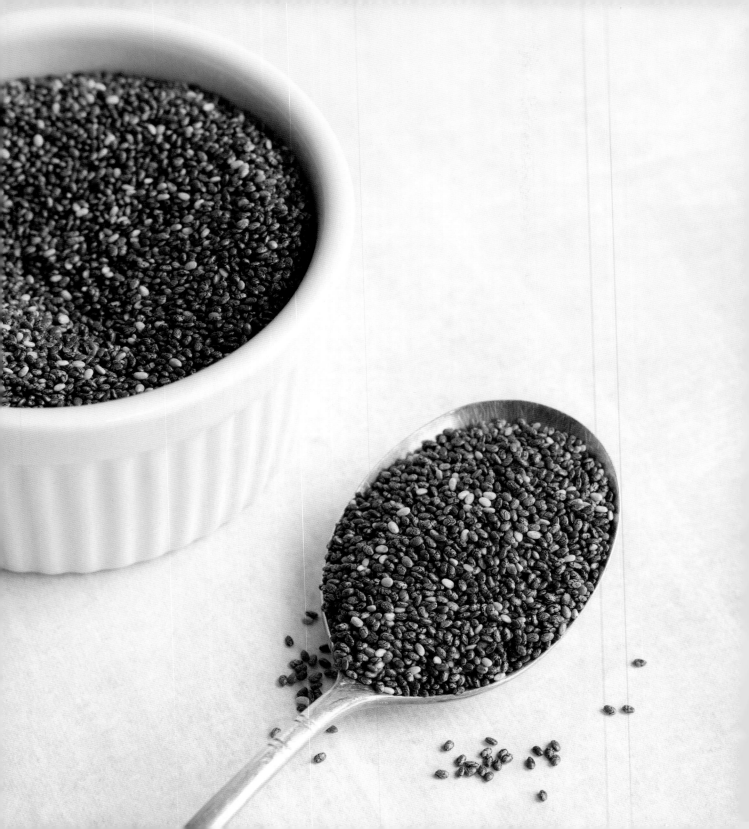

# the
## essentials

Let's dive in and learn how to create plant-based versions of pantry staples—from dairy substitutes, such as coconut yogurt (page 55), nut and seed milk (pages 50 and 52) and Cheesy Kale Chips (page 64) to mouthwatering sauerkraut (page 67), Date Syrup (page 56) and more. This section is here to help you avoid pricey store-bought and processed vegan alternatives and still enjoy nutritious, exciting food at every meal.

# pure nut mylk

Raw | alkalizing | protein rich  •  Soaking time: overnight | Yields: 3 cups (710 ml)

We have been making homemade nut mylk for years now, and we encourage you to do the same. I know you might think that getting a box of almond milk from a store is just so much more convenient, but have you ever looked at the ingredients? It's rather long and a bit scary! Do we really need guar gum, carrageenan and lecithin? In general, these additives are mostly preservatives, thickeners and stabilizers, homogenizing the mixture and thickening it to more resemble cow's milk. Without these additives, nut milk will separate. But you know what? All you have to do is shake it. This homemade nut mylk has only two ingredients—raw nuts and purified water. Not only is homemade nut mylk delicious, but it goes great in your morning warm drinks, smoothies, tonics and even dressings!

1 cup (140 g) raw, unsalted nuts (almonds, hazelnuts, Brazil nuts, pecans, macadamias, walnuts)

3 cups (710 ml) purified water for blending, plus more if desired

Soak the nuts overnight in 2 to 3 cups (475 to 710 ml) of water.

Drain and discard the soaking water and rinse the nuts well. Place the nuts in a blender along with the 3 cups (710 ml) of purified water. Blend on high speed for 2 to 3 minutes, or until smooth.

Strain the blended nut mixture through a cheesecloth or a nut milk bag, squeezing out as much liquid as possible.

If you want a thinner nut mylk, add more purified water as desired.

Pour into a glass jar and refrigerate. The mylk will keep in the refrigerator for 3 to 4 days.

## pro tips:

•   The easiest possible nut mylk to make is from cashews. The softness of the nut means there is barely any pulp. You could even get away without straining the mylk if you are okay with a slightly gritty texture.

•   Removing the skins from almonds gives them a smooth texture, which is helpful in such recipes as this. To begin, soak your almonds for 2 hours or overnight, drain and rinse well. Use your fingers to gently squeeze the almonds and loosen the skin from them. Be careful; if you squeeze too hard, they'll shoot across the room—which is fun, but not practical! Once all the almonds are peeled, rinse them again and they'll be blanched and ready to use in the recipe.

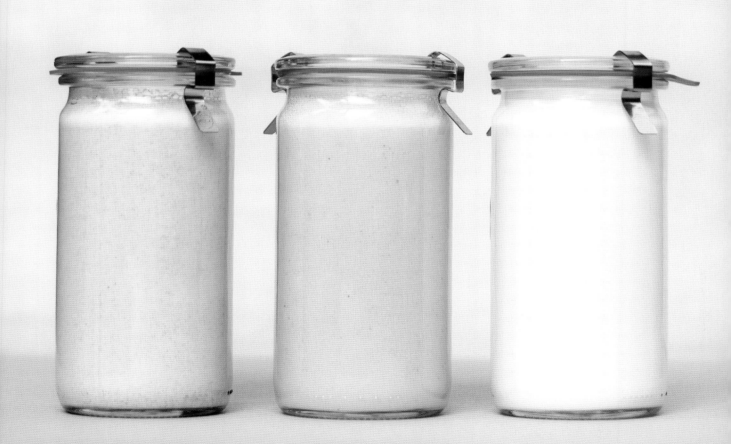

# hemp mylk

Raw | complete protein | skin and hair strengthener    •    Yields: 3 cups (710 ml)

If you want a convenient, fast and delicious plant-based mylk for smoothies, chia puddings and nourishing warm drinks, then hemp mylk is the way to go! Not only is it easy to make, but hemp mylk is a nutritional powerhouse. Hemp hearts are high in complete protein, abundant in essential fatty acids as well as calcium and iron. We have added dates and cinnamon to this recipe to balance the pronounced flavor of hemp; however, feel free to adjust the ingredients to suit your taste.

½ cup (90 g) hemp hearts

3 cups (710 ml) purified water, for blending

½ tsp ground cinnamon

2 dates, pitted

In a blender, combine all the ingredients and blend until smooth and creamy.

Pour into a glass jar with a tight lid and refrigerate. Your hemp mylk will last for up to 5 days in the fridge.

*See photo on page 51.

**note:**

This mylk is best to use within the first two days. After that, it still remains tasty; however, you might find that it separates or curdles if you add it to your warm beverage. It's best to use in smoothies after a few days.

**pro tip:**

If you prefer a smoother texture, then take the extra step to strain the hemp mylk through a nut milk bag or cheesecloth. Do not discard the pulp as there are still lots of nutrients left. Instead, add the pulp to your smoothies or dressings.

# quinoa mylk

Alkalizing | bone strengthener | complete protein  •  Soaking time: overnight | Yields: 4 cups (946 ml)

Did you know you can make mylk from quinoa? It's a straightforward and nutrient-dense, plant-based dairy alternative that's hugely beneficial to your active life. Quinoa is an excellent source of protein and contains the eight essential amino acids, so it's a perfect food for muscle growth. It's gluten-free, has a low glycemic index, is high in fiber, regulates cholesterol levels, prevents constipation and is rich in essential fatty acids (omega-3 and omega-6), B vitamins, iron and potassium. When you use this quinoa mylk as the base for your smoothies, you will seriously up your game. Give it a try and see for yourself.

½ cup (87 g) uncooked quinoa

4 cups (946 ml) purified water, for blending

4 dates

Soak the quinoa overnight in 1 cup (240 ml) of water. Before cooking, drain through a fine strainer and rinse until the water runs clear.

To cook, in a medium saucepan, bring another 2 cups (475 ml) of water to a boil. Add the quinoa and bring to a second boil, then cover and simmer over low heat for 15 minutes. Remove from the heat and allow the quinoa to cool. Place the cooled quinoa in a blender with the 4 cups (946 ml) of purified water. Blend on high speed for 1 to 3 minutes, or until smooth.

Strain the blended quinoa mixture, using a cheesecloth or a nut milk bag. The milk will strain through slowly on its own, but you can gently squeeze and massage the bottom of the cloth to speed up the process.

Pour the quinoa mylk back in the blender, add the dates and blend until smooth.

Transfer the quinoa mylk to a glass jar with a tight lid and store in the fridge for 3 to 4 days.

*See photo on page 51.

## pro tip:

Quinoa is naturally coated in a bitter resin called saponin that deters birds and insects from eating the seed. Saponin must be removed by carefully rinsing the quinoa to make it palatable. Most of the saponin will have been removed before the quinoa was shipped to the store, but there will likely be a powdery residue. Simply follow the instructions in this recipe to ensure great-tasting quinoa mylk.

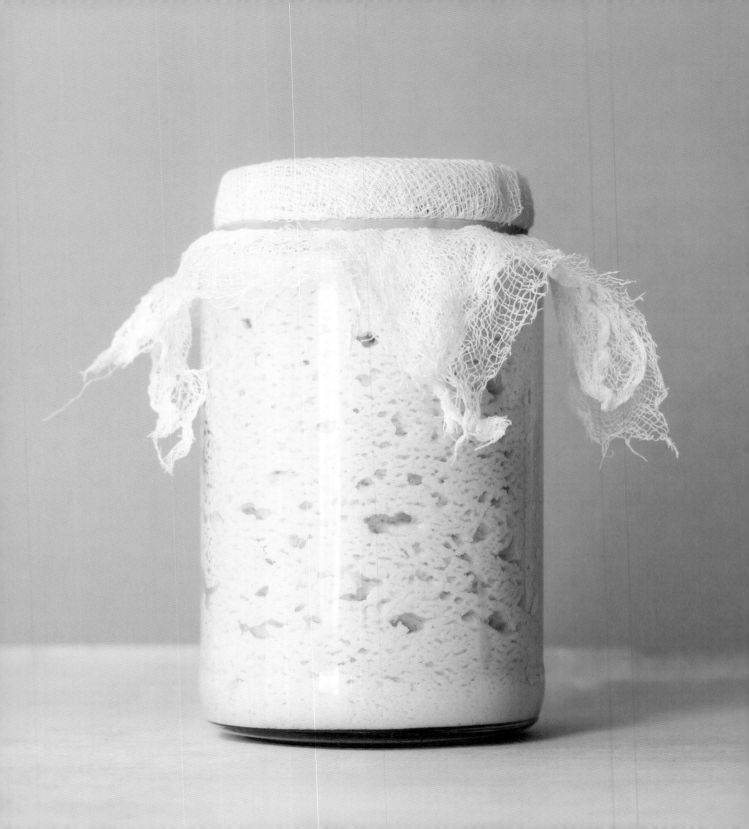

# cultured coconut yogurt

Raw | digestive aid | protein rich  •  Yields: 1 quart (1 L)

We've been making coconut yogurt for a while now. It's a staple in our diet, supersimple to make and very beneficial for gut health. At the time of writing this book, there are just a few nondairy yogurt brands available at the supermarkets here in Canada. However, they all include thickeners and additives, such as carrageenan, locust bean gum, guar gum, sugar, "natural" flavors and other ingredients! On the other hand, our recipe has only three (that's right, three) ingredients. The result is nothing short of amazing. The texture is thick and silky. The taste is a bit tangy and sour with a hint of coconut—just like a yogurt ought to be. Eat it plain, top it with fresh or dried fruit, add it to your smoothie bowls and chia puddings, use it as a base in a creamy sauce or simply sprinkle it with granola!

2 cups (1 lb [455 g]) young Thai coconut meat (1 to 4 coconuts)

¼ to ½ cup (60 to 120 ml) coconut water (depending on preferred thickness)

2 capsules probiotics (see notes)

In a high-speed blender, combine the coconut meat and coconut water and blend until very smooth. Make sure you blend it long enough to get a creamy texture because it won't get any smoother as it ferments.

Add the powder from the 2 capsules of probiotics (discard the capsules) and blend again for only a few seconds until combined.

Transfer the mixture to a 1-quart (1-L) glass mason jar, making sure to fill it no more than three-quarters full. Doing this allows for expansion. Cover with a cheesecloth and fasten the cloth with a rubber band.

Place in a dark, warm space for 24 hours. We put ours in the kitchen cupboard. Taste as it ferments. You might like it strong tasting or not. Note also that the fermenting process speeds up in warmer temperatures.

Store your yogurt, sealed with a tight lid, in the fridge. It should last for 5 days.

## pro tips:

- Make sure that all your utensils and the jar you ferment with are extremely clean.
- Do not use metal utensils as they will disrupt the fermentation.

### notes:

- If you don't like coconut or can't find fresh coconuts, you can use 2 cups (280 g) of soaked, then drained, raw cashews instead.
- There are tons of different probiotics out there, so don't get overwhelmed. The probiotic that we currently use for fermentation is Natren Megadophilus Dairy Free Capsules, available at most natural food stores. However, you can use any brand that you have on hand.

# date syrup

Raw | antioxidant rich | low glycemic    •    Soaking time: 30 minutes | Yields: 1⅓ cups (320 ml)

Talk about fast, easy and healthy. Date syrup is a great staple to keep handy in your fridge. This whole-food, natural sweetener is low-glycemic, rich in antioxidants and high in vitamins and such minerals as potassium and magnesium, and it's very versatile. You can use it to sweeten your morning drinks or nut mylks, drizzle it on top of smoothie bowls or coconut yogurt and also use it in baked recipes as a replacement for other syrups made with high-fructose corn syrup or other processed sugars. Dates are cholesterol-free and low-fat. They are a good source of protein and dietary fiber and are rich in vitamins $B_1$, $B_2$, $B_3$ and $B_5$ along with $A_1$ and C. They are known to help improve the digestive system, as dates contain soluble and insoluble fiber and a variety of amino acids. Want a quick and natural energy boost before your run? A couple of spoonfuls of this date syrup will do the trick!

1 cup (178 g) Medjool dates, pitted (about 10 large dates)

1¼ cups (295 ml) purified water, for blending

1½ tsp (8 ml) fresh lemon juice

In a small bowl, cover the dates with warm water (not the purified water) and let sit for 30 minutes.

Drain and rinse the dates. Place them in a high-speed blender together with the purified water and lemon juice. Blend for 45 to 60 seconds, or until smooth.

Transfer to an airtight container and store in the refrigerator for up to 2 weeks.

## serving suggestions:

*   Drizzle over pancakes and waffles.

*   Add to smoothies.

*   Drizzle over smoothie bowls, quinoa porridge or chia pudding.

*   Use in baking and for making power bars.

*   Use as a sweetener to replace any other sweetener; for example, add to your tea, nut mylks, health tonics, etc.

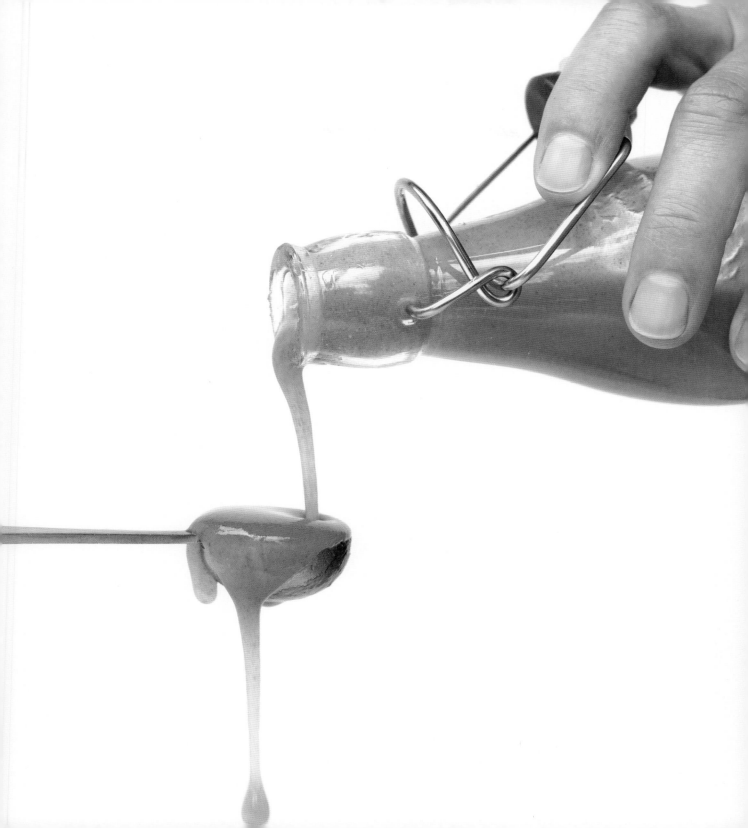

# power nut butter

Raw | supports healthy heart | protein rich • Soaking time: 8+ hours (optional) | Yields: 1½ cups (390 g)

Fresh homemade nut butter is a treat few can resist. It's a satisfying and very convenient food that is good to always have on hand. This nut butter is made with maca and cinnamon, which help boost energy and stamina, combat fatigue and regulate blood sugar. For a quick and easy protein boost, add a spoonful to your smoothie, drizzle some over coconut yogurt or spread onto anything from lettuce wraps to sprouted-grain toast.

1½ cups (218 g) raw almonds

1 cup (100 g) raw walnuts

½ cup (90 g) hemp hearts

1 tsp maca powder (optional)

1 tsp ground cinnamon

Pinch of Celtic sea salt

If sprouting your nuts, follow the instructions in the pro tip.

In a processor or high-powered blender, combine the almonds, walnuts and hemp hearts. Blend on medium-low speed until creamy, 8 to 10 minutes, pausing to scrape down the sides as necessary.

Add the maca (if using), cinnamon and salt. Blend until thoroughly incorporated.

Transfer the nut butter to a glass jar with a tight-fitting lid. Store in the fridge and enjoy within a few weeks.

## pro tip:

Up the nutritional value by sprouting the almonds and walnuts prior to using:

Soak the nuts in water to cover, along with ½ teaspoon of salt, for 8 hours or overnight. Drain and rinse, then dry the nuts in an oven or dehydrator.

To oven dry, set the oven to the lowest possible temperature. Spread out the nuts on an ungreased baking sheet and bake with the door ajar for 2 to 3 hours, or until bone dry and crispy, tossing every hour.

If using a dehydrator, spread on the mesh sheet and dry for 8 to 12 hours at 110°F (43°C) until crispy and dry, tossing halfway through.

# green mix salad

Raw | alkalizing | calcium & iron rich   •   Yields: 2 servings

This salad is a staple of the Plant-Powered Diet. Include at least one big serving of greens in your daily meals. The basic mix is made from a variety of dark leafy greens that offer a fiber-rich source of carbohydrates, an excellent source of calcium and a variety of vitamins and minerals—all important for a healthy athlete. We suggest you always have a container of this mix on hand as it makes a great start to a fantastic meal.

1 head romaine lettuce, chopped

2 cups (40 g) baby arugula

1 cup (30 g) baby spinach

1 cup (40 g) fresh cilantro, chopped

1 cup (60 g) fresh parsley, chopped

In a big salad bowl, combine all the greens. Eat fresh or store in a closed container in the fridge for 2 to 3 days.

*See photo on page 61.

**note:**

Mix and match with a variety of seasonal ingredients and top it with any dressings, dips or sauces from this book. Be creative; the possibilities are endless.

**pro tip:**

Incorporating greens into your diet doesn't have to be a challenge. Try adding a handful of this mix to every meal, including your smoothies.

# superfood salad topper

Raw | protein packed | high in antioxidants　•　Yields: 2⅓ cups (337 g)

Obviously, we love salad and enjoy making it pretty much daily. To keep things interesting, we often look for ways to up our salad game and give our meals an extra nutritional boost. One way to achieve this is by adding different superfoods to the mix. So, that is how the superfood salad topper came to life. It's a flavorful, nutrient-dense mix of chia, flax, hemp hearts, pumpkin, sunflower and sesame seeds, raw cashews, goji berries and spices. It takes only five minutes to put together and will give your salads a major boost of flavorful protein crunch.

½ cup (70 g) raw cashews

½ cup (70 g) sprouted or raw pumpkin seeds

1 cup (160 g) mixed seeds (sunflower, chia, flax, hemp)

⅓ cup (37 g) goji berries

2 tbsp (30 ml) flax oil or extra virgin olive oil

1 tsp curry powder

1 tsp ground turmeric

½ tsp ground cinnamon

Pinch of cayenne pepper

Pinch of sea salt

In a large bowl, combine the nuts, seeds and goji berries and toss with the oil, curry powder, turmeric, cinnamon, cayenne and salt.

Ideally, allow the mix to marinate for 15 minutes before serving.

Store the mixture in an airtight glass container in the fridge or freezer. It will keep fresh for weeks, ready to quickly nourish your meals.

> **note:**
>
> Add this mix to your salads or quinoa bowl or sprinkle on top of soup. It also makes a great quick snack on its own.

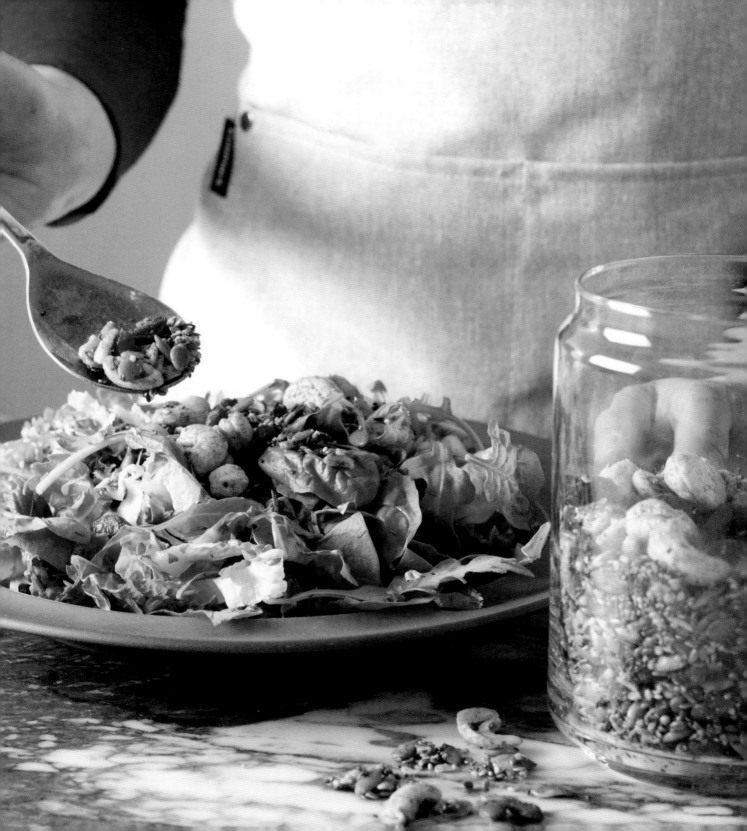

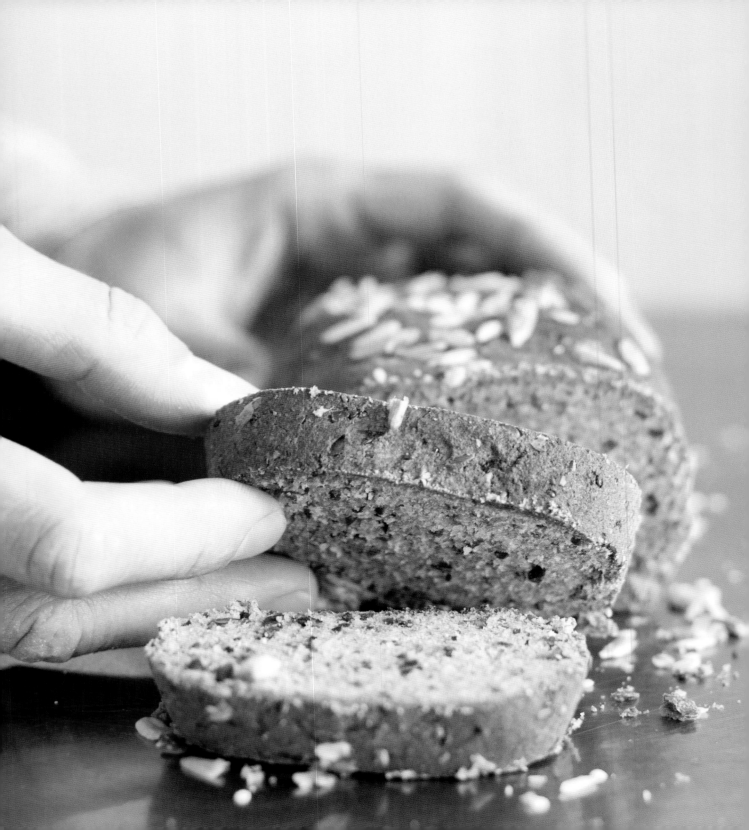

# simple nut & seed bread

Protein rich | supports repair and recovery  •  Soaking time: 4+ hours | Yields: 10 slices

This is a simple recipe for a grain-free, protein-rich, nut and seed bread that you can easily make in your kitchen. However, before we dive into how to prepare it, let me share with you why I chose some of the ingredients. The moist almond pulp gives the bread a lovely light texture, plus it is a great way to upcycle the leftover pulp from your homemade almond mylk. Psyllium husk provides this bread with a spongy texture that is otherwise challenging to accomplish with grain-free bread. Also, the combo of flax, hemp and chia seeds is a real nutritional powerhouse. The essential fatty acids found in these seeds provide the fuel that our body needs to function more efficiently, thereby reducing stress. Overall, this is a fantastic staple in your plant-powered kitchen and so easy to make!

1 cup (145 g) almonds, soaked in water for 4 hours or overnight

½ cup (73 g) sunflower seeds, soaked in water for 4 hours or overnight

½ cup (89 g) pitted dates

¼ cup (42 g) flaxseeds

¼ cup (20 g) whole psyllium husk

¼ cup (44 g) hemp hearts

1½ tbsp (15 g) chia seeds

½ cup (80 g) chopped onion

2 cloves garlic

1 tsp Himalayan pink salt

Unsoaked sunflower seeds, sesame seeds or your choice of topping

Drain the soaked almonds and sunflower seeds, rinse and dry very well.

In a food processor fitted with the S blade, combine all the ingredients, except the toppings, and blend until everything is incorporated. You may need to stop a few times and scrape down the sides with a spatula.

Transfer to a cutting board and press the mixture together until it is evenly combined and compact.

Form the dough into a loaf or your preferred shape and coat the top with extra sunflower seeds, sesame seeds or your choice of topping.

**baked**
Preheat your oven to 350°F (180°C). Place the loaf on a baking sheet lined with a piece of parchment paper. Bake for 40 to 50 minutes, or until a toothpick inserted into the center comes out clean. Remove from the oven and let the bread cool down completely before cutting into it. When it is ready to serve, use a serrated knife to cut it.

**raw**
Dehydrate at 145°F (63°C) for 1 hour. This will create a crust on the outside. Remove the bread and place on a cutting board. Using a serrated knife, cut the bread into ½- to 1-inch (1.3- to 2.5-cm)-thick slices. It's helpful to clean the knife in between cuts to make each cut nice and even. Lay each slice, cut side down, on the mesh sheet. Decrease the temperature to 115°F (46°C) and continue to dehydrate for 4 to 6 hours.

Store the bread in a tightly sealed container for up to 5 days. It freezes well too.

# cheesy kale chips

Bone support | anti-inflammatory   •   Soaking time: 2+ hours | Yields: 2 cups (100 g)

These chips are real powerhouses of nutrition and also crunchy and satisfying. Per calorie, kale provides more nutrients than any other vegetable on the planet. It contains dozens of minerals, antioxidants and phytonutrients, including vitamins A, C and K. One cup (67 g) of kale, which would make a small serving of kale chips, contains 472 micrograms of vitamin $K_1$, which makes it the perfect choice for fighting inflammation and providing cardiovascular support. Enjoy these chips as a midafternoon snack or sprinkled on your salad.

½ cup (73 g) raw sunflower seeds, soaked in water for at least 2 hours or overnight

⅓ cup (43 g) nutritional yeast

2 tbsp (30 ml) raw cider vinegar

¼ tsp ground turmeric

1 clove garlic

⅓ tsp sea salt

4 cups (268 g) curly kale

1½ tsp (8 ml) extra virgin olive oil

Preheat the oven to 275°F (140°C) or set a dehydrator to 115°F (46°C). If oven baking, line 2 baking sheets with parchment paper.

In a food processor or blender, combine the sunflower seeds, nutritional yeast, cider vinegar, turmeric, garlic and salt. Blend until well mixed. If your mixture is very thick, add a little drizzle of water to make it more manageable when massaging onto the kale. Set aside.

Wash your kale thoroughly. Use a paper towel or clean dish towel to completely dry the kale. Tear or cut the kale leaves off their stem and rip them into chip-sized pieces.

Place the leaves in a large bowl, drizzle with the olive oil and using your hands massage the oil thoroughly all over the leaves. Add a generous amount of the cheesy paste and gently massage it through the leaves as evenly as you can.

### baked
Spread out the kale leaves in a single layer on your prepared baking sheet, separating them so they'll cook quickly and stay crunchy.

Bake for 12 to 15 minutes, checking occasionally. Remove from the oven and flip them over. Bake for another 5 to 10 minutes, or until just crunchy but still green.

### raw
Spread out the leaves on the mesh sheets of a dehydrator and dehydrate at 110°F (43°C) for about 8 hours (overnight or while you're at work).

Kale chips are best when fresh; however, you can store them in an airtight container for 2 to 4 days.

### pro tip:
Leftover cheesy sauce can be used as a salad dressing. Just mix in 1 to 2 tablespoons (15 to 30 ml) of purified water to thin it out.

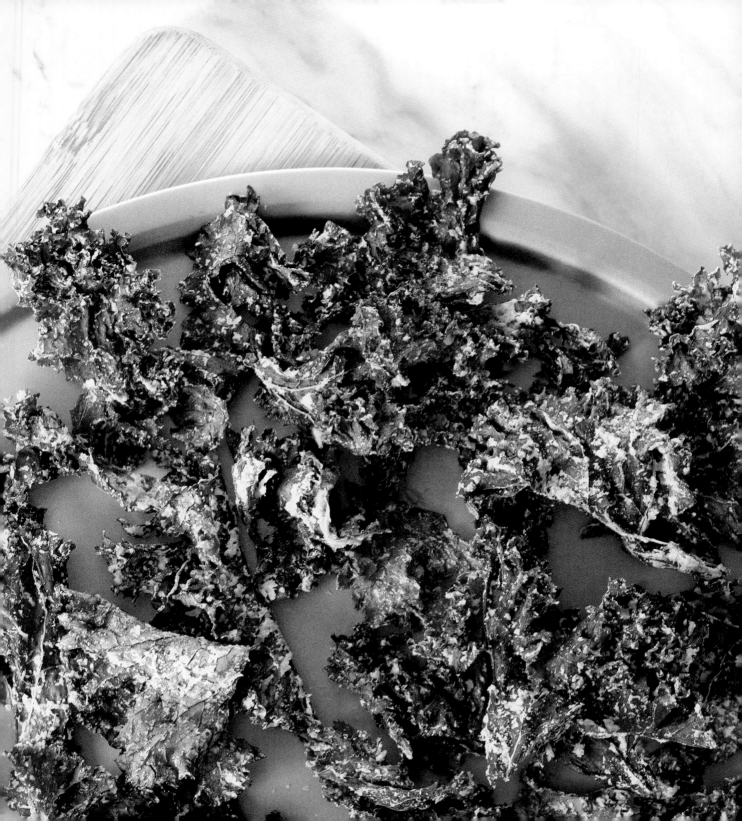

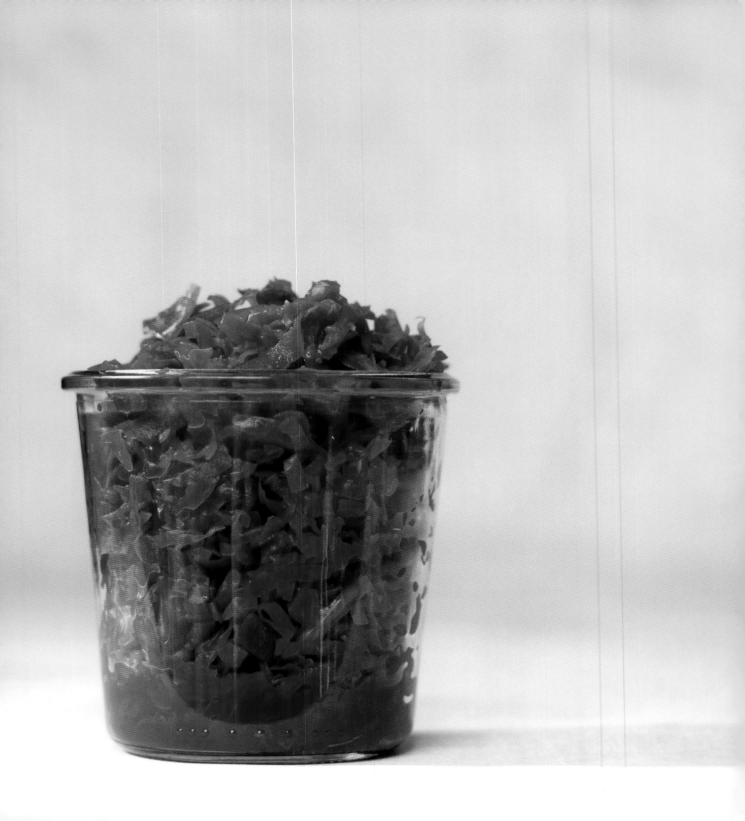

# gut-healing sauerkraut

Raw | packed with probiotics | vitamin C rich    •    Yields: 4 cups (568 g)

Including cultured foods like this raw sauerkraut in your diet can make a massive difference in the way you digest food, the way you feel and the overall health of your body. If you are new to fermenting and feel a bit hesitant, we hope to put your mind at ease. Take a deep breath and give this recipe a try. Honestly, making sauerkraut at home is supersimple. Organic cabbages are easy to get—and inexpensive! You don't need any special equipment and it only takes a few days to ferment a small batch of incredibly delicious probiotic-rich sauerkraut!

1 medium purple cabbage (908 g)

1 tbsp (13 g) Celtic sea salt (see notes)

2 to 4 tbsp (28 to 56 g) minced fresh ginger, to taste (optional; see notes)

## notes:

- Salt choice is significant with fermented foods. You want to avoid processed salts, such as table salt and iodized salt, as they contain additives that can inhibit fermentation. Your best salt choices are those that are fine grained, dry and mineral rich, such as Celtic sea salt or Himalayan pink salt.

- The amount of ginger you will want to add is totally up to you. The smaller amount will create a kraut with a more subtle gingery note, and the larger amount will give the kraut more of a spicy kick.

Peel off and discard any wrinkly, dry or damaged outer leaves from the cabbage. Reserving 1 healthy, pliable leaf for later, cut the cabbage into quarters right through the core. Carefully cut out and discard the tough inner core. Shred the cabbage, using a mandoline, knife or food processor. We prefer using a food processor fitted with the shredding blade.

Put the shredded cabbage into a large bowl. Sprinkle the salt over the cabbage and massage it with your hands until liquid starts to release. Set aside to marinate.

Add the minced ginger to the bowl of cabbage. Use your hands to work the ginger through the cabbage evenly, then once again massage the cabbage until it releases plenty of liquid when squeezed in your hands. The released juice will later be used as a brine.

Transfer the cabbage to a wide-mouth 1-quart (1-L) mason jar, packing it down tightly with each handful added to the jar. When the cabbage is tightly packed down, take the cabbage leaf you reserved earlier and gently fold it until it is about the same width all around as the jar. Place the leaf into the jar, on top of the packed cabbage and make sure it covers it completely.

Press the cabbage leaf down firmly, then pour enough brine from the mixing bowl to cover all of the cabbage and submerge it in the liquid. The cabbage must be below the water (brine) level, away from oxygen. Be sure to leave an inch (2.5 cm) of space between the top of liquid and the top of the jar. Doing this allows for expansion. However, do not leave too much room at the top of the jar as too much oxygen could cause your kraut to go bad.

Allow the kraut to ferment in a cool, dark place for at least 3 days and up to 10, depending on your desired degree of sourness. Once the kraut has fermented to your liking, seal the jar and transfer it to the refrigerator. Fermenting will continue to take place in the fridge, but this will be very, very slow. The flavors may change over time.

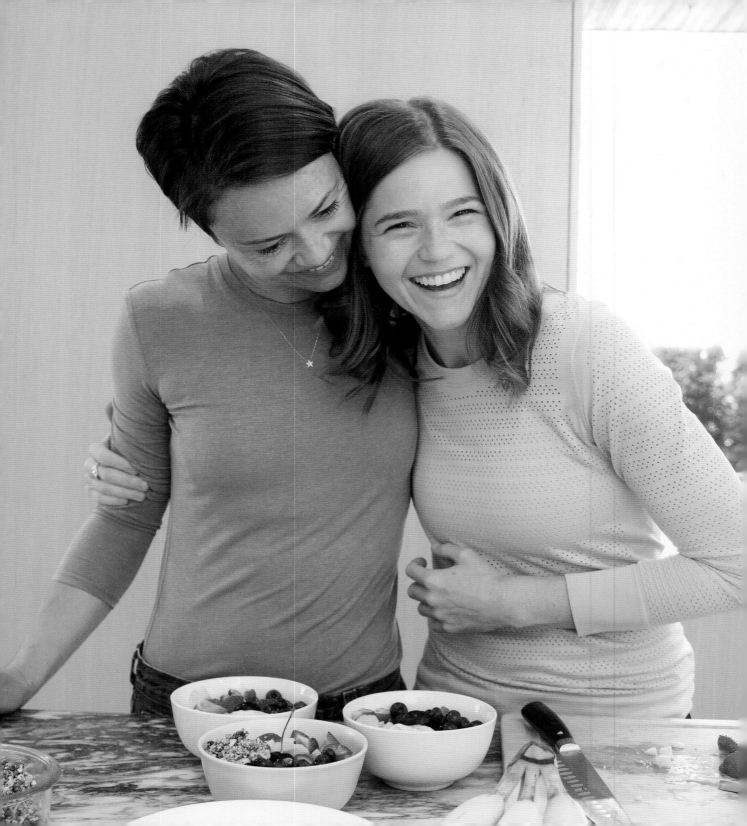

# healthy start

Whether you break your fast first thing in the morning or much later in the day, your first meal should deliver the energy and nutrients you need to perform at your best. If you want to train like an athlete, or aspire to look like one, eating like one is a great place to start. With such recipes as the Powerhouse Green Juice (page 72), 5-Minute Raw Granola (page 88) or Spinach Crepes (page 93), this healthy start lineup has you covered—whether you're looking for a high-energy postworkout recharge, a grab-and-go smoothie or a leisurely weekend brunch.

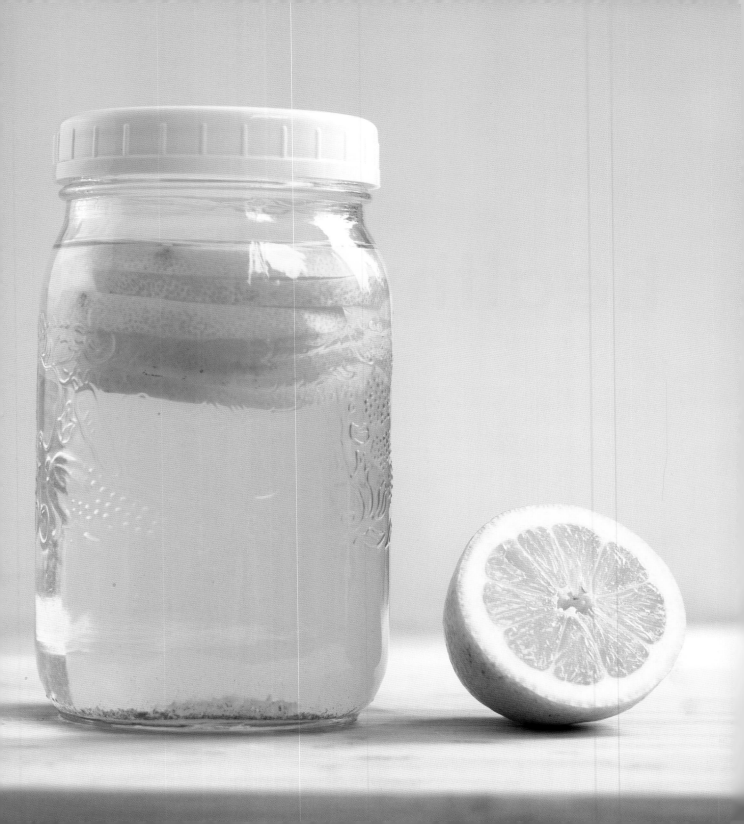

# cleansing morning lemonade

Raw | detoxifying | immunity booster  •  Yields: 1 quart (1 L)

Get into a habit of drinking one glass of warm water after rising. Doing this will help to end the "drought" of the night and help regulate bowel movement. Then, drink a second glass of warm water, this time made with fresh lemon juice, a teaspoon of raw agave and a pinch of cayenne pepper—we call it the Morning Lemonade. This drink helps stimulate the liver (the main detoxifying organ in the body) and flush out old waste and harmful bacteria from the gastrointestinal tract, leaving you feeling light and refreshed!

1 large lemon

1 quart (1 L) warm purified water

Pinch of cayenne pepper, or to taste

1 to 2 tsp (5 to 10 ml) raw agave nectar (optional)

Wash the lemon well and squeeze the juice into a 1-quart (1-L) glass or mason jar. Add the purified water, cayenne and agave (if using).

Stir and drink first thing in the morning on an empty stomach.

> **note:**
>
> In the spring and summer months, we like to make the recipe using cold purified water. In the fall and winter months, we use warm water instead. Experiment to learn what you like best.

# powerhouse green juice

Raw | protein rich | cleansing  •  Yields: 1 serving

Green juice is a staple at our house mostly because it's tasty, quick and filled to the brim with powerhouse ingredients! This juice is loaded with chlorophyll, which strengthens red blood cells and in turn naturally boosts energy levels. This juice is also very energizing. It will help increase your ability to tackle the day without the need for caffeine and rid you of an after-lunch productivity drop.

4 ribs celery

6 sprigs flat-leaf parsley (leaves and tender stems)

2 packed cups (65 g) spinach leaves

6 seasonal green leaves (collard leaves, lettuce leaves, kale, Swiss chard, etc.)

3 green apples, cored and chopped

½ lemon, peeled

1 (1" [2.5-cm]) piece fresh ginger

Process all the ingredients through a juicer, alternating between hard and soft items.

**note:**

Try to drink your juice immediately. After 15 minutes, light and air will destroy many of the nutrients. If you can't drink it fresh, transfer it to an airtight glass container until you're ready.

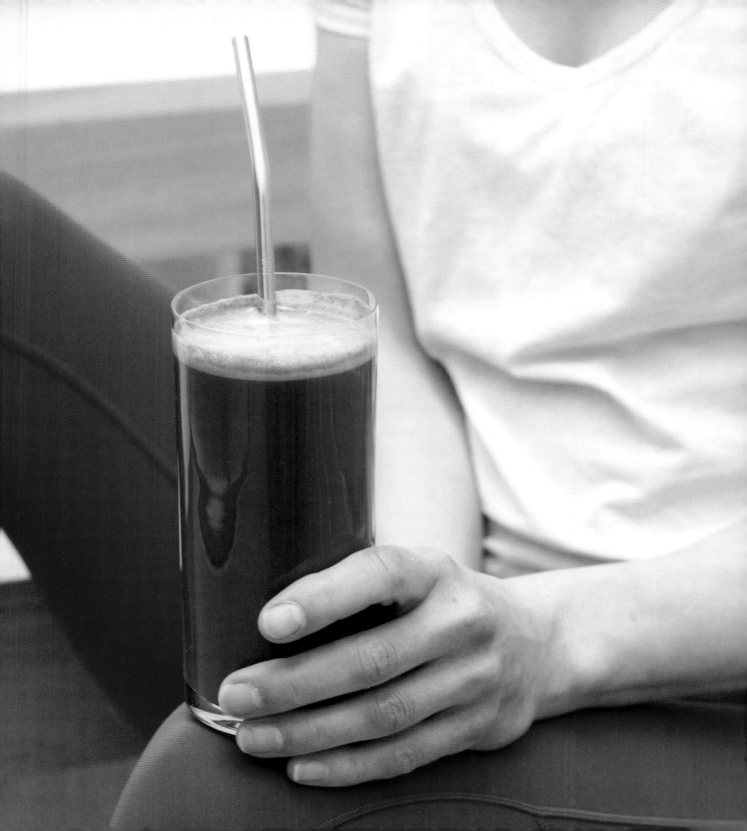

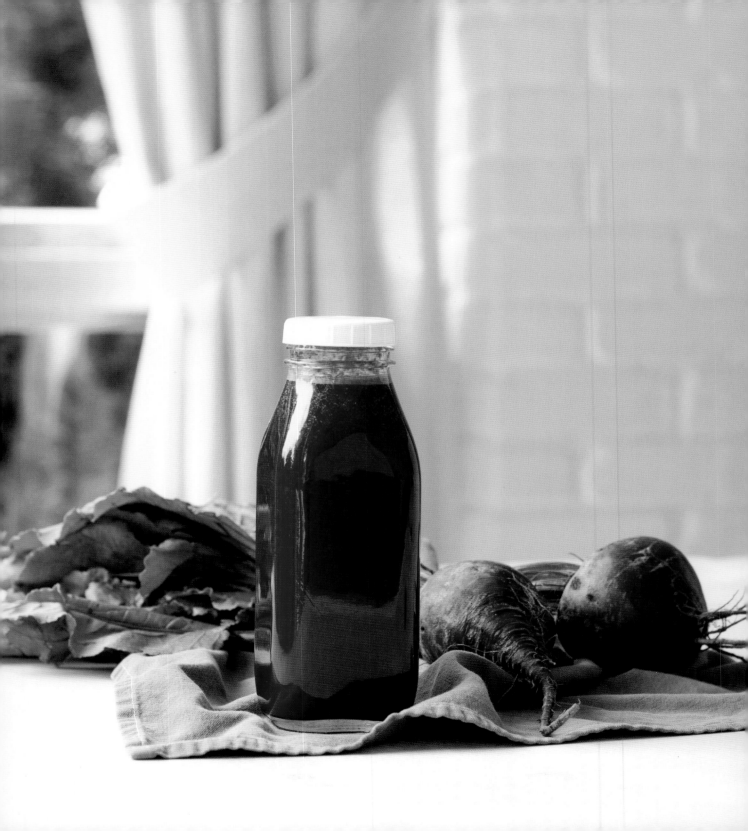

# liver flush juice

Raw | fat flushing | detoxifying  •  Yields: 1 serving

A perfect health tonic that supports the immune system, lowers swelling and elevates your overall health and performance. Why liver flush? Well, because the liver is one of the hardest-working organs in the body. It works tirelessly to detoxify your blood, produce the bile needed to digest fat, break down hormones and store essential vitamins and minerals. Unfortunately, most people struggle with an overburdened liver, due to a toxic diet and lifestyle. In consequence, their body is ineffective at digestion and breaking down fat, resulting in weight gain and in feeling heavy, bloated and sluggish. Juicing is a powerful way to support the cleansing of your liver without compromising your body's natural healing process. This is one of our favorite juice combinations that contain unique antioxidants and anti-inflammatory nutrients to help with the detoxification process, nourish your liver cells and support their regeneration.

1 beet, scrubbed and trimmed

1 (1″ [2.5-cm]) piece fresh turmeric, or 1 tsp ground turmeric

5 carrots, scrubbed and trimmed

1 grapefruit, peeled

1 lemon, peeled

¼ cup (60 ml) purified water, if using a blender

**using a juicer**
Put all the ingredients through your juicer. Stir and serve immediately.

**without a juicer**
Cut the vegetables into bite-sized pieces.

In a blender, combine all the ingredients and blend until smooth, adding about ¼ cup (60 ml) of purified water. Place a fine-mesh strainer over a large bowl and pour the juice through. Use a wooden spoon or spatula to press the pulp down and squeeze out all the juice. Allow to sit for 2 to 3 minutes to let most of the juice drain. Discard the pulp and pour your juice into a serving glass. Drink immediately.

# rise 'n' shine smoothie

Raw | energizing | anti-inflammatory  •  Yields: 1 serving

This smoothie is an energizing breakfast or preworkout meal. Pineapple combined with jalapeño, an excellent metabolism booster, and cucumber creates this simple, refreshing smoothie that will have you going strong for hours. Hemp hearts are a rich source of protein and give this "liquid meal" a smooth, creamy texture. Unlike many traditional breakfasts, this one digests easily, giving you the ability to think clearly and work efficiently for hours.

1 cup (240 ml) purified water

1 cup (165 g) fresh or frozen pineapple chunks

1 cup (135 g) chopped cucumber

Large handful of baby spinach

1 to 3 slices jalapeño pepper, seeds removed (or more to taste)

1 tbsp (11 g) hemp hearts

Pinch of Celtic sea salt (optional)

In a blender, combine all the ingredients and blend on high speed until smooth, 10 to 20 seconds. Serve immediately.

**note:**

This smoothie has a spicy kick—adjust the jalapeño quantity to give it just the right amount of spice you desire.

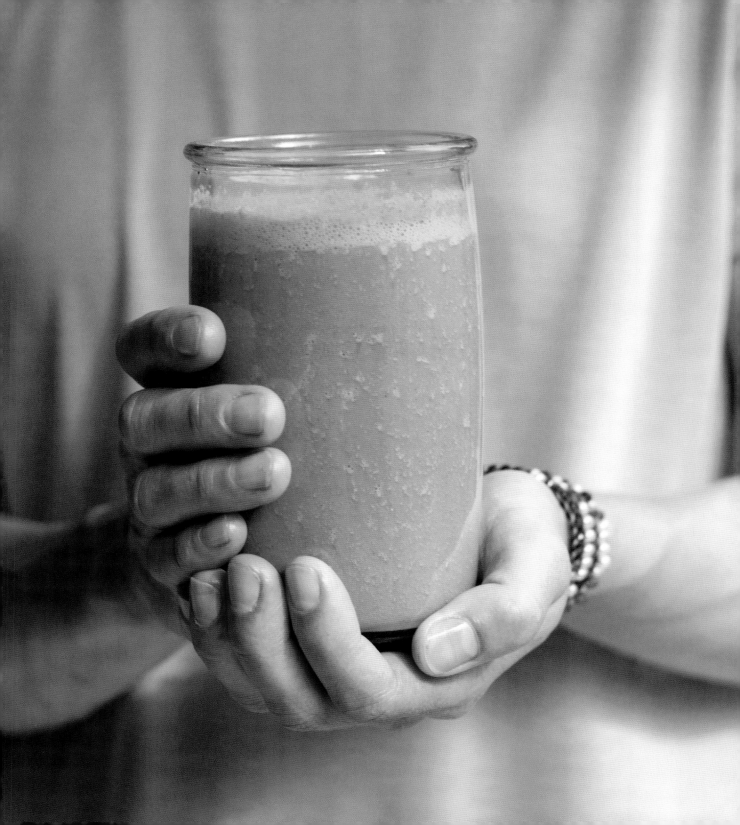

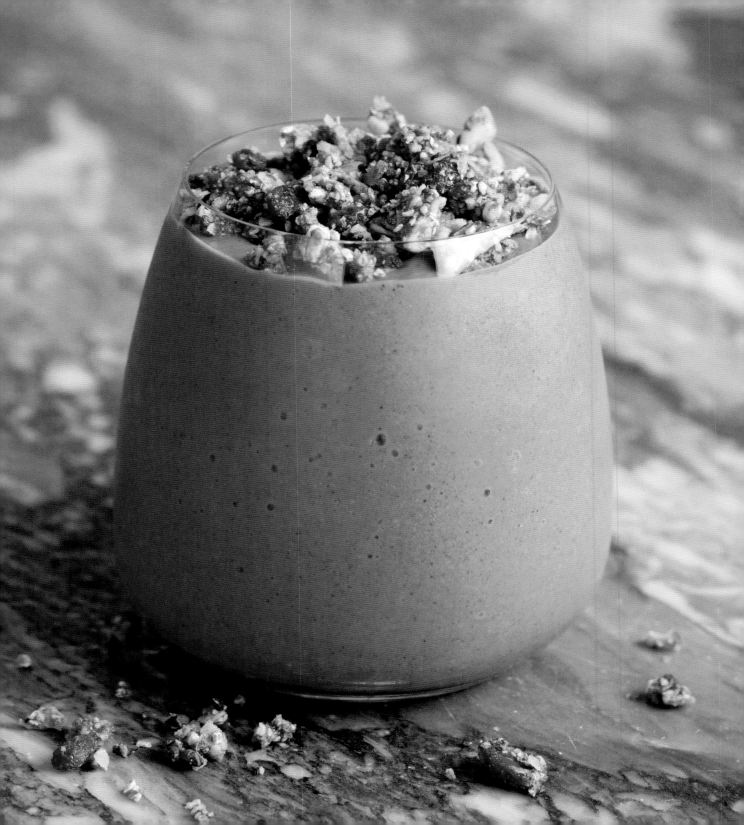

# morning energizer smoothie

Raw | high in antioxidants | protein rich  •  Yields: 1 serving

It's a great habit to include a nutritious smoothie in your diet every day, and this one is designed to keep you going through your busy day. The combination of ingredients will ensure your body gets all the nourishment it needs from living whole food sources. Plus, starting your day with a liquid meal will help take the strain off your digestive system, therefore providing you with higher energy. It's also an excellent choice for preworkout fuel.

1 cup (240 ml) purified water

1 fresh or frozen banana

1 cup (120 g) chopped zucchini

2 tbsp (13 g) goji berries

1 tsp maca powder

4 Brazil nuts

1 tbsp (10 g) chia seeds

1 tbsp (8 g) hemp protein powder

1 tbsp (7 g) raw cacao powder

2 tbsp (13 g) 5-Minute Raw Granola (page 88; optional)

In a blender, combine all the ingredients, except the granola, and blend until smooth.

If you want to make the smoothie into a more substantial meal, you can top it with 2 tablespoons (13 g) of the raw granola.

**note:**

Use carob instead of cacao for a no-caffeine alternative.

**pro tip:**

Try to drink your smoothie immediately. After 15 minutes, light and air will destroy many of the nutrients. If you can't drink it fresh, transfer it to a dark, airtight container and store in the fridge until you're ready.

# matcha latte

Raw | energizing | high in antioxidants  •  Yields: 1 serving

This latte with homemade nut mylk is not only supereasy to make, but it also tastes better than anything you would get in a fancy coffee shop. The highlight of this blend is the powerful source of matcha, which has been consumed for centuries to promote detoxification, concentration and high energy levels. The addition of coconut butter and dates makes this latte a perfect breakfast, snack or meal replacement that will keep you full for hours, promote mental clarity and increase fat burning. We suggest that you take the extra five minutes to make homemade plant-based mylk (pages 50 to 53). It is easy, and makes the latte so much creamier and tastier.

1 cup (240 ml) plant-based mylk (pages 50–53; almond or hemp works great)

⅓ cup (80 ml) hot water

1 to 2 Medjool dates, pitted

1 tsp matcha powder

¼ tsp raw vanilla powder or ground cinnamon

1 tbsp (15 g) coconut butter or oil

### high-speed blender method

In a high-speed blender, combine all the ingredients and blast on high speed for 3 to 4 minutes, or until the mixture gets nicely heated.

### stovetop method

If you don't have a high-speed blender yet, here is what you do: In a conventional blender, blend all the ingredients on high speed for 20 seconds, or until the matcha has been incorporated evenly, and transfer to a small pot. Gently warm over medium-low heat (do not boil) for a few minutes, until hot.

### note:

When purchasing matcha powder, look for quality over quantity. Matcha powder should be certified USDA Organic and stored in a sealed, airtight container.

### pro tip:

Matcha contains caffeine, a nerve toxin that stimulates the adrenal glands to secrete stress hormones and trigger an immune response that may give you a sense of energy and vitality. Sometimes, lightly stimulating foods, such as matcha, can be consumed to yield a significant boost in athletic performance. However, afterward, it is important to take appropriate steps to recover from this extra adrenal stimulation. In other words, regular use of caffeine will have a decreased impact on the body. Please do not rely on caffeine day after day; instead, use it as an occasional treat.

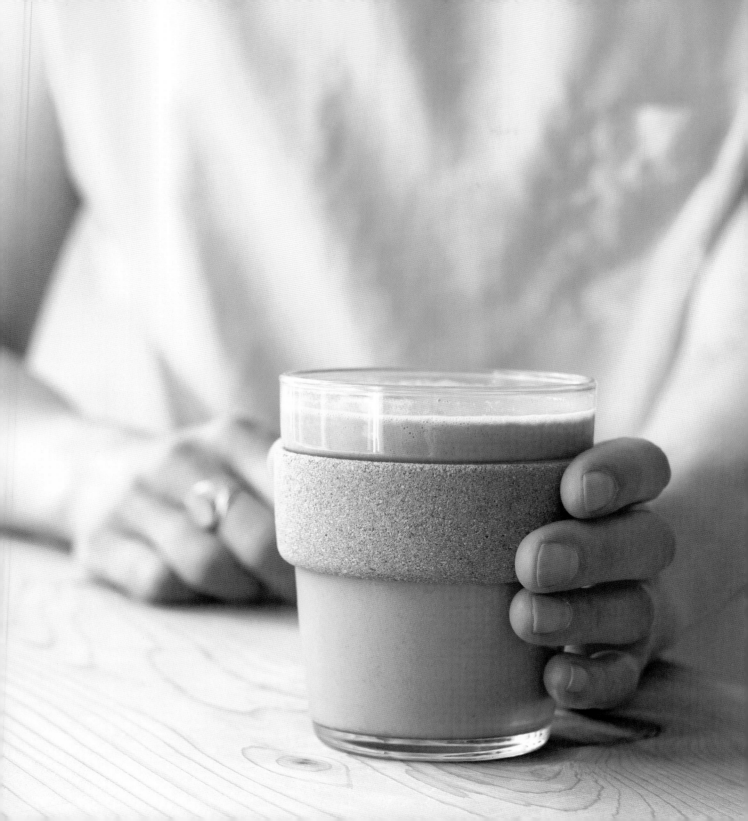

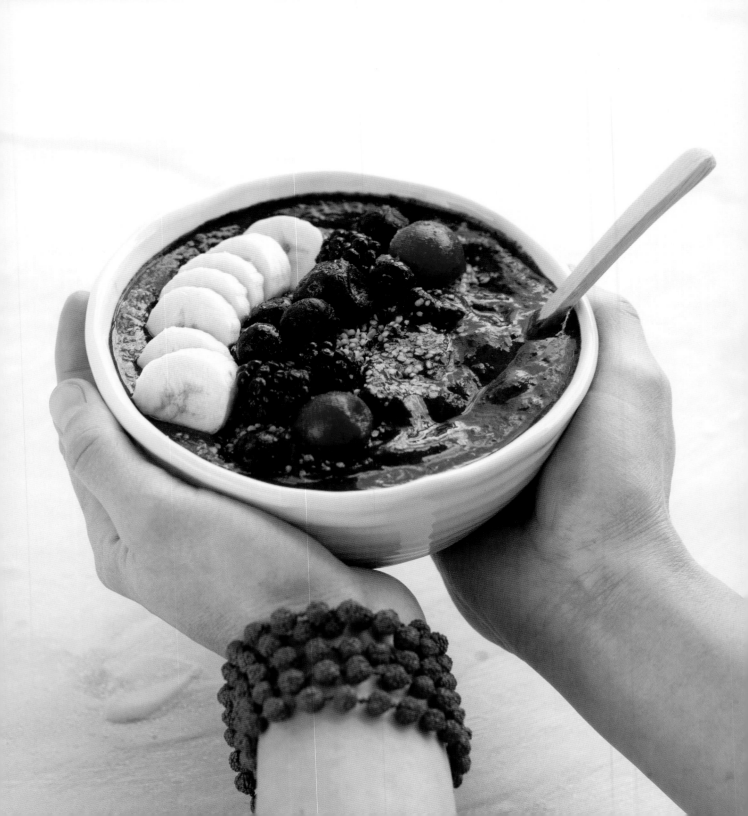

# maqui berry smoothie bowl

Raw | high in antioxidants | brain boosting  •  Yields: 1 serving

This smoothie bowl is a nutrient bomb. Made with frozen berries, spinach, bananas and maqui berry powder, it's a great option for breakfast if you're used to having regular smoothies in the morning. Ethically grown berries of all varieties are a superfood packed with fiber, potassium, vitamin C, folate and a host of other phytonutrients that keep us healthy, vibrant and glowing. Maqui berry powder (from the Chilean dried fruit) is a highly concentrated source of antioxidants that help prevent free radical damage and slow the aging process. This smoothie bowl also contains vitamins A, C and E; essential minerals, such as calcium, iron and potassium; and anti-inflammatory compounds. Feel free to top with your favorite nuts, seeds and superfoods.

1½ frozen bananas

1 cup (150 g) frozen berries of your choice

Big handful of baby spinach

1 Medjool date, pitted

½ cup (120 ml) plant-based mylk (pages 50–53; almond or hemp works great)

2 tbsp (24 g) hemp protein powder

1 tsp maqui powder

½ tsp raw vanilla powder

Pinch of Himalayan pink salt

**topping suggestions**

Fresh berries

Fresh banana

Fresh mango

Sunflower seeds

Pumpkin seeds

Chia seeds

Shredded unsweetened coconut

Sprouted buckwheat

Macadamia nuts

In a high-speed blender, combine all the ingredients, except the toppings, and blend until smooth.

Scoop the mixture into a bowl and garnish with your toppings of choice.

Eat immediately!

# carrot cake smoothie bowl

Raw | anti-inflammatory | muscle meal  •  Yields: 1 serving

This creamy smoothie bowl is a healthy, simple spin off classic carrot cake. It makes a perfect breakfast choice, especially after a good morning workout. The beta-carotene from carrots helps fight free radicals that build up during exercise, and the coconut yogurt is full of amino acids (particularly threonine), beneficial for building healthy connective tissues as well as speeding up your recovery. Also included are turmeric, ginger and pineapple, all containing potent anti-inflammatory compounds that help soothe pain and inflammation.

Overall, this is a great meal to help you nourish and recover after a good training session.

1 cup (186 g) frozen pineapple

1 large carrot, chopped

2 dates, pitted

¼ cup (60 g) Cultured Coconut Yogurt (page 55) or coconut cream

½ tsp ground turmeric

1 (1″ [2.5-cm]) piece fresh ginger, peeled

¼ tsp ground cinnamon

## topping suggestions

Shredded unsweetened coconut

Fresh berries

Fresh herbs

Chia seeds

Mulberries

Pistachios

Nut butter

Additional yogurt

Walnuts

Ground cinnamon

In a high-powered blender, combine all the ingredients, except the toppings, and blend until smooth.

Add your toppings of choice.

**variations:**

Alternatively, you could swap in a different type of fruit for the natural sweetness. Mango, apple or pear would all work well.

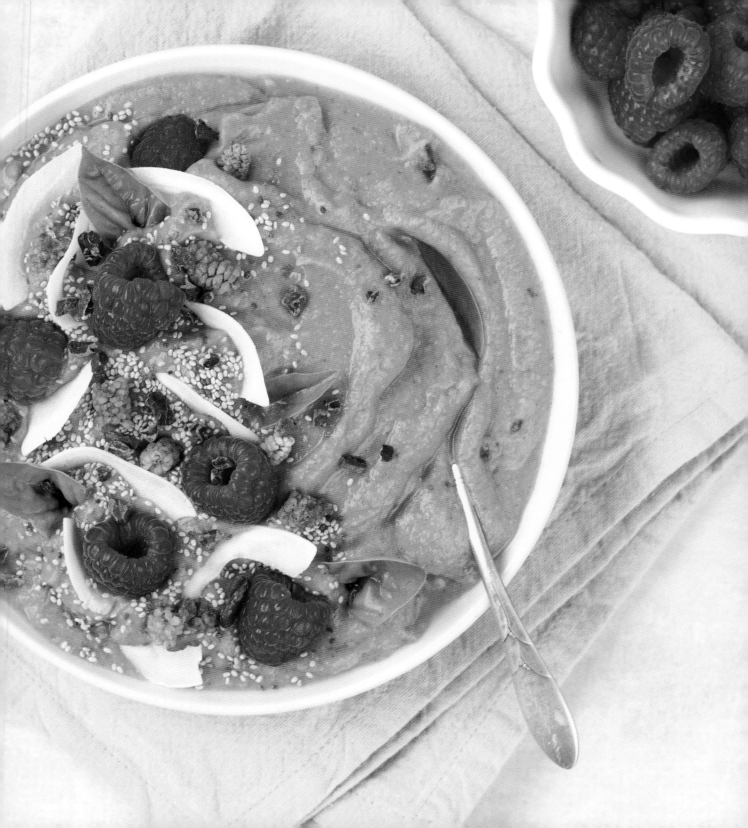

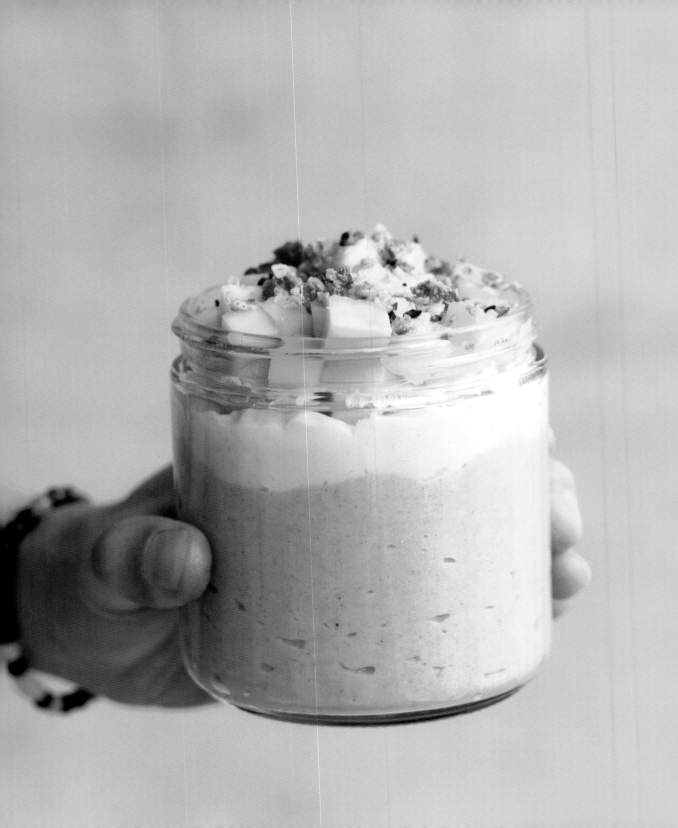

# creamy mango-chia pudding

Raw | protein & mineral rich | energizing  •  Yields: 2 servings

This recipe is quite versatile: Want to enjoy it for breakfast? It's a quick porridge. Crave a dessert? Here is a sweet pudding for you. Want it for a snack? Call it "My Preworkout Warrior Food." Seriously, though, there are many great things to say about the ingredients used in this recipe, but let's narrow it down to just two. Mangoes are one of our favorite fruits. They are sweet, juicy and packed full of goodness—antioxidants, fiber, folate, vitamin C and a hefty dose of vitamin A that keep your eyes and bones healthy. Chia seeds are pretty magical athlete's fuel, because of their ability to increase stamina and sustain energy over long periods. They also help prevent dehydration, are alkalizing to the body and rich in omega-3 fatty acids and provide a healthy dose of dietary fiber. On top of that, chia seeds are also chock-full of antioxidants, contain high-quality complete protein, are low-glycemic and will also provide you with antioxidants, calcium, omega-6, phosphorous, magnesium, iron and zinc. Now, that's an impressive high-density nutrient meal!

## mango-chia pudding

1 cup (240 ml) almond mylk (page 50)

1 cup (175 g) peeled and chopped fresh or frozen mango

1½ tsp (8 g) maca powder

¼ cup (40 g) chia seeds

2 tbsp (30 ml) fresh lime juice

2 dates, pitted

1 (½" [1.3-cm]) piece fresh ginger, peeled

## topping suggestions (optional)

Cultured Coconut Yogurt (page 55)

Fresh fruit

5-Minute Raw Granola (page 88)

Shredded unsweetened coconut

Prepare the pudding: In a high-speed blender or food processor, combine all the pudding ingredients. Blend on high speed until smooth.

Divide between 2 jars and place in the fridge. Allow the mixture to sit for 20 minutes so the chia seeds can thicken everything up.

You can enjoy it as is or serve it with your desired toppings.

Any leftover chia pudding can be stored in an airtight container in the fridge for up to 3 days.

**notes:**

- Adjust the amount of ginger to your personal preference.

- The possibilities are endless here: You can use different fruits and/or plant-based mylks and change up your toppings, too.

# 5-minute raw granola

Raw | protein rich | energizing • Yields: 2 cups (200 g)

Granola is such a convenient food, whether you enjoy it for breakfast, a snack or as a topping, you really can't go wrong with having some around. Unfortunately, most store-bought kinds are loaded with refined sugars, processed oils and artificial flavors. For that reason, we encourage you to make your own. This raw granola takes only a few minutes to make; it's naturally sweet, made with a variety of sun-dried fruits, seeds and coconut flakes. No artificial flavors. No added colors. Just the taste you love and the nutrition you want.

¼ cup (35 g) raisins

¼ cup (28 g) dried mulberries

1 cup (85 g) unsweetened large coconut flakes

¼ cup (35 g) pumpkin seeds

¼ cup (36 g) sesame seeds

½ tsp ground cinnamon

¼ tsp raw vanilla powder

Pinch of sea salt

Rinse and drain the raisins and mulberries.

In a blender or food processor, combine all the ingredients. Pulse on low speed until everything is combined. If using a blender, you may have to shake the blender a few times if it gets stuck.

Store in an airtight container in the fridge for up to 5 days.

## serving suggestions:

- Enjoy it as a quick breakfast with some plant-based mylk (pages 50–53) or Cultured Coconut Yogurt (page 55).
- Sprinkle a couple of spoonfuls on top of your smoothie bowl for a nice crunch.

## pro tips:

- This is not a crunchy granola. It's soft, with a chewy texture. If you want a little crunch, feel free to mix in some nuts of your choice or cacao nibs.
- To keep this granola fully raw, use unhulled sesame seeds (i.e., in the shell). Unhulled sesame seeds are very crunchy, almost hard, and taste slightly bitter. Toasted hulled sesame seeds (not raw), on the other hand, have a nutty, clean flavor.

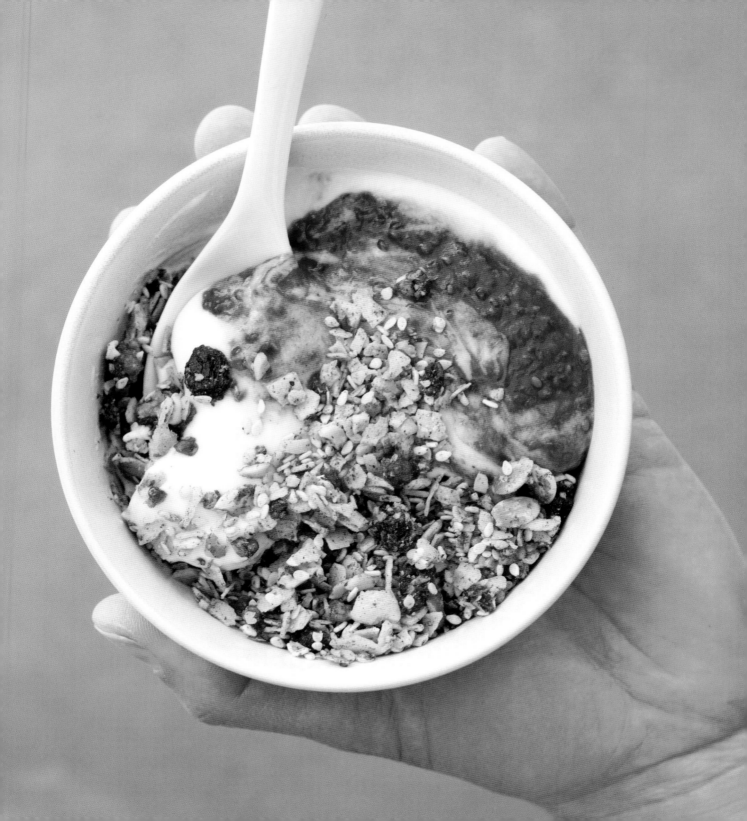

# avocado & pea smash

Raw | muscle meal | postworkout recovery  •  Yields: 1 serving

This one-bowl-only pea smash is so simple, and it requires only essential ingredients that you probably already have in your fridge. The combination of green peas and avocado creates quite the nutritional powerhouse; you are nourishing yourself with healthy fats, the right amount of protein, fiber and plenty of vitamin C. Also, avocado is one of the best sources of potassium—an important mineral for athletes as it helps maintain electrolyte balance, prevents cramping and reduces blood pressure. Enjoy this smash on toast, with fresh-cut veggies or on the side of a large green salad.

¼ cup (35 g) fresh or frozen peas

½ medium avocado, peeled and pitted (see notes)

1 tbsp (15 ml) fresh lime juice

¼ tsp Celtic sea salt

¼ cup (10 g) fresh herbs, such as basil, mint or cilantro, chopped

**to serve**

2 slices sprouted-grain bread, a wrap (such as Ezekiel brand) or flax crackers (optional)

Fresh-cut veggies (optional)

Sprouts, for garnish (optional)

If using frozen peas, place in a glass cup or bowl and cover with hot water. Set aside for 5 minutes.

Meanwhile, scoop the avocado into a medium bowl. Add the lime juice and salt, then mash together with a fork until a creamy consistency is achieved.

Drain the defrosted peas and add them (or the fresh peas) to the avocado bowl together with your herbs of choice. Mix well.

Serve on a slice of sprouted-grain bread, in a wrap, on flax crackers or in a bowl with fresh-cut veggies. Garnish with sprouts (if using).

**notes:**

- This smash is best served fresh, or within 30 minutes of making.

- If you plan on making it for next-day lunch, put it in a small glass container with limited space on top, insert the avocado pit into the pea smash, seal and place in the fridge. The flavor will remain and the pit will keep the avocado from turning brown.

# smoky tempeh scramble

Muscle building | post workout recovery | calcium rich • Yields: 1 or 2 servings

This simple-to-prepare savory morning meal, full of protein and veggies, could easily pass for lunch or dinner. Tempeh is a fantastic plant-based source of easy-to-digest protein that has a delicious nutty flavor and satisfying taste. It's also very high in magnesium and is known to reduce cholesterol, increase bone density and promote muscle recovery. This recipe is excellent on its own; however, if you prefer a heartier meal, feel free to serve it on top of avocado, along with some greens; wrap it up into a burrito; or eat it with sprouted-grain toast. For anyone who is looking to build muscle, this tempeh scramble could be a real game changer.

1½ tsp (8 ml) extra virgin coconut oil

1 clove garlic, minced

¼ cup (40 g) diced onion

½ red bell pepper, seeded and diced

½ cup (84 g) crumbled tempeh

¼ tsp ground turmeric

¼ tsp smoked paprika

Celtic sea salt

Freshly ground black pepper

1 cup (30 g) baby spinach, chopped

2 tbsp (8 g) fresh parsley, chopped

Heat a small nonstick skillet over medium heat.

Add the coconut oil and once hot and simmering, add the garlic and onion. Sauté for 1 minute. Add the bell pepper and sauté for 2 minutes. Add the tempeh, turmeric, smoked paprika, salt and black pepper to taste; stir to combine.

Cook, stirring, until the tempeh is hot and evenly coated in the seasoning mixture, 3 minutes. Add the spinach and parsley and sauté for 1 more minute. Taste the tempeh scramble and season with more spices as desired.

Serve on its own, on top of sprouted-grain bread, wrapped in a tortilla or alongside of Green Mix Salad (page 59) or an avocado.

note:

Don't be scared to add more veggies if you got them! This would also be fabulous with zucchini, asparagus, mushrooms, etc.

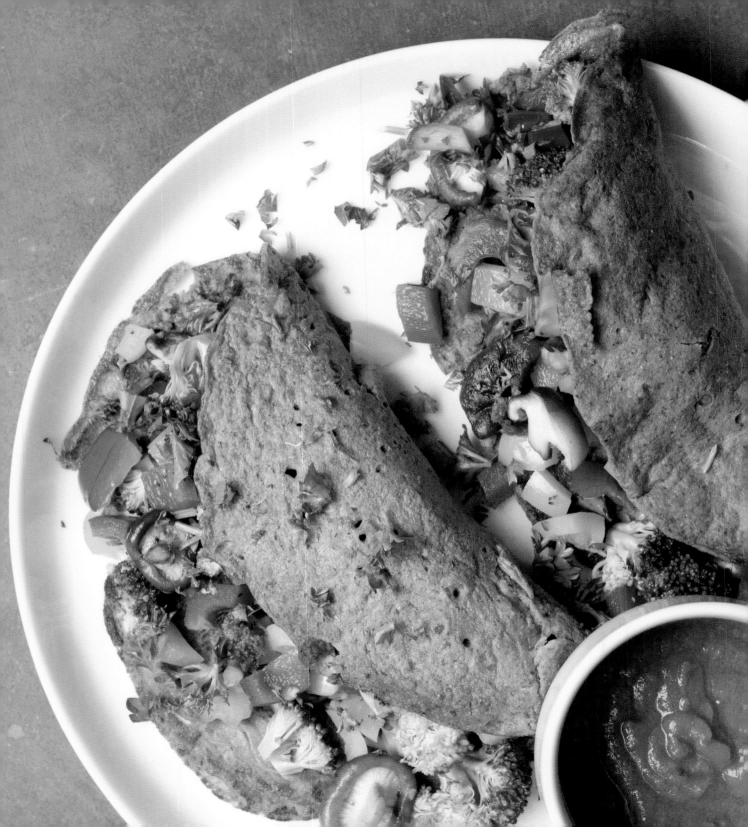

# spinach crepes

Muscle building | iron rich | high fiber  •  Yields: 2 crepes

Don't be intimidated by making crepes—they are much easier than you might think! These spinach crepes take about 20 minutes to prepare and miraculously don't fall apart or stick to the pan, despite the absence of eggs and oil in the batter. Spinach is a source of iron; chickpea (garbanzo) flour provides steady energy and, though once a rarity, is now commonly available in supermarkets. This recipe is filling, a perfect choice for a postworkout morning meal or Sunday brunch with friends and family. The spinach taste is mild, so if you are still a bit apprehensive about making these crepes, don't be! Give them a try!

½ cup (120 g) chickpea flour

1 tsp ground flaxseeds

¾ cup (175 ml) water

2 handfuls of spinach

Celtic sea salt and freshly ground black pepper

1 tsp coconut oil, divided, for frying

Your choice of fillings—our personal favorites are sautéed mushrooms, bell peppers, cherry tomatoes, fresh herbs, avocado and Cilantro Chutney (page 201)

In a blender, combine the chickpea flour, flaxseeds, water, spinach, salt and pepper to taste and blitz for a few minutes, until everything is well combined. Let the batter rest for 5 to 10 minutes.

In a 7-inch (18-cm) skillet, heat ½ teaspoon coconut oil over medium heat. Add ¼ cup (60 ml) of the batter to the pan and swirl around the bottom so you get an even crepe.

Cook over medium heat for about 2 minutes, or until there are bubbles in the crepe and you can lift it up to easily flip it.

Flip and cook on the other side for 30 seconds to 1 minute.

Remove from the pan, place on a plate and cover with a clean cloth to keep warm.

Repeat the process with the rest of the oil and batter.

Stuff the crepes with your choice of fillings.

## pro tips:

- To make successful crepes, you have to start with the right batter consistency. You should be able to quickly spread the batter around the pan and make thin pancakes, lightly crisped up around the edges.

- Crepe batter that's too thick will not spread as easily and will yield thicker pancakes. If your batter is a little too thick, add a drop of water to it.

- You can make small or large crepes, depending on personal preference. It's generally easier to make smaller crepes.

- It's also important to lightly oil the pan and cook the crepes over medium heat. I use about ½ teaspoon of coconut oil per crepe and oil the pan using a pastry brush or small piece of paper towel.

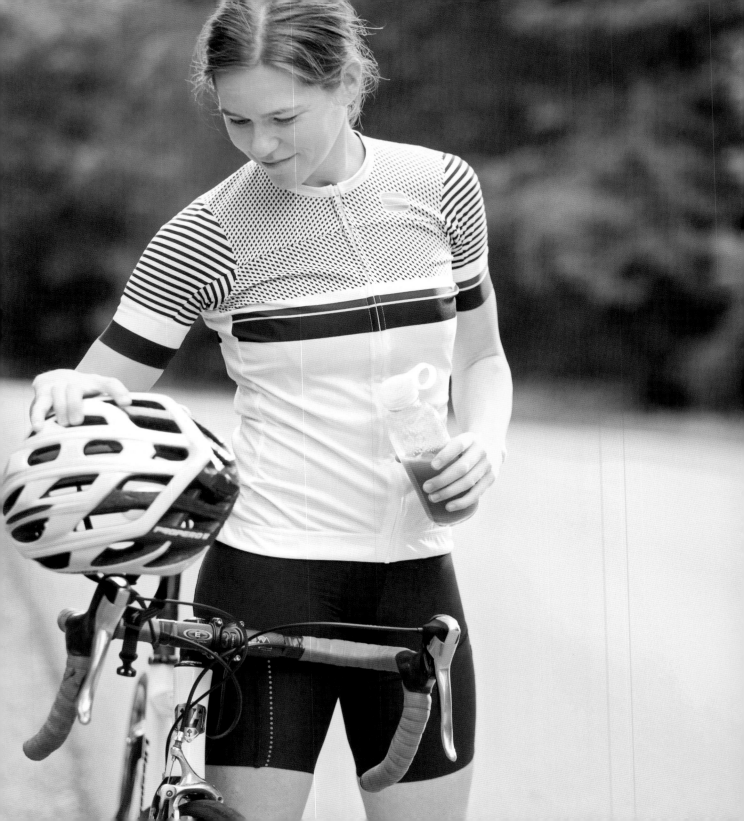

# workout fuel

The most efficient way to achieve your fitness goals is through effective training combined with optimal nutrition. We have tested and used the following simple plant-powered recipes over the years to fuel our performance, build strength and speed up recovery. Included are packable Coco-Mango Performance Bars (page 122) that will nourish you throughout the day, preworkout Cucumber-Lime Chia Fresca (page 96), postworkout Chocolate Muscle Mylk (page 112), endurance gels (pages 117 and 118) and plenty of other nutrient-dense ideas to keep you on top of your game.

# cucumber-lime chia fresca

Raw | hydrating | sustained energy  •  Yields: 2 cups (475 ml)

This refreshing drink is a perfect morning preworkout rehydrator. It's a combination of three wonderful foods that help replenish the significant water loss that happens during nighttime rest. Chia seeds, cucumbers and coconut water are all deeply hydrating, replenishing and nourishing to the body from the inside out. Mixing these creates a beverage rich in electrolytes, omega-3s, protein and fiber. This mixture can also serve as an energy drink during a longer, sweaty workout.

½ large cucumber, coarsely chopped

2 cups (475 ml) coconut water or purified water

Juice of 1 small lime

1 tbsp (15 ml) raw agave nectar or Date Syrup (page 56)

1 tbsp (10 g) chia seeds

In a blender, combine the cucumber, coconut water, lime juice and agave. Blend until smooth.

Pour the mixture through a fine-mesh strainer fitted over a small bowl. Press the juice pulp against the strainer to extract as much liquid as possible. Discard the pulp.

Transfer the juice to a big glass jar or pitcher and add the chia seeds. Stir well and allow to sit for at least 10 minutes in the fridge while the chia seeds swell. After the seeds expand, they like to sink to the bottom of the jar. That's no problem—just be sure to give the drink a nice stir or shake before you drink it.

Store in the fridge and enjoy within 2 to 3 days.

**note:**

Whenever possible, use fresh, unprocessed coconut water from a young Thai coconut. If unavailable, replace the coconut water with purified water.

**pro tip:**

To get the most juice out of a lime, before cutting it, roll the whole lime back and forth on the counter while pressing down firmly. Rolling like this for about 10 seconds will help loosen up the juices inside.

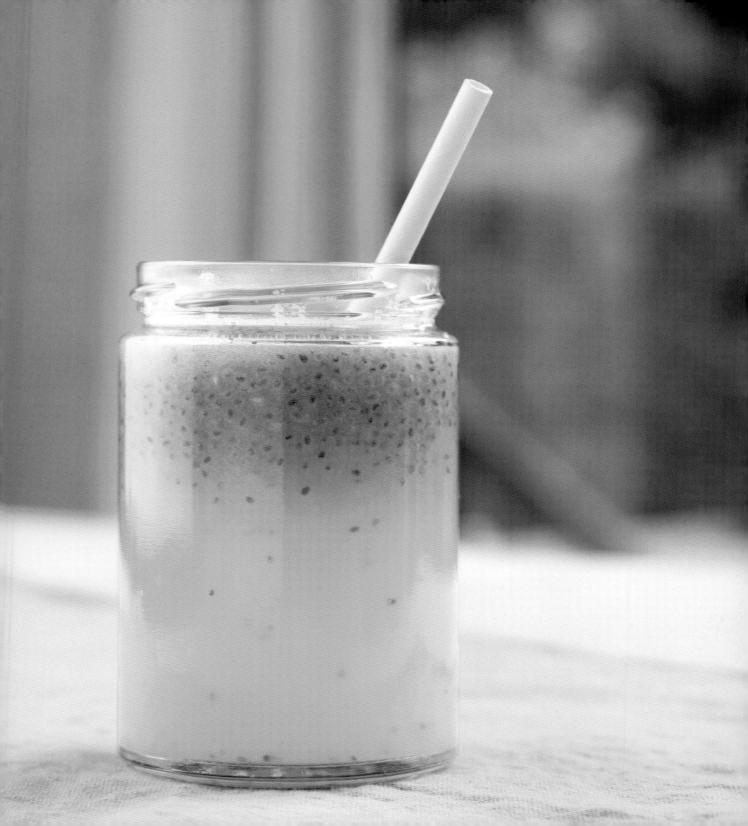

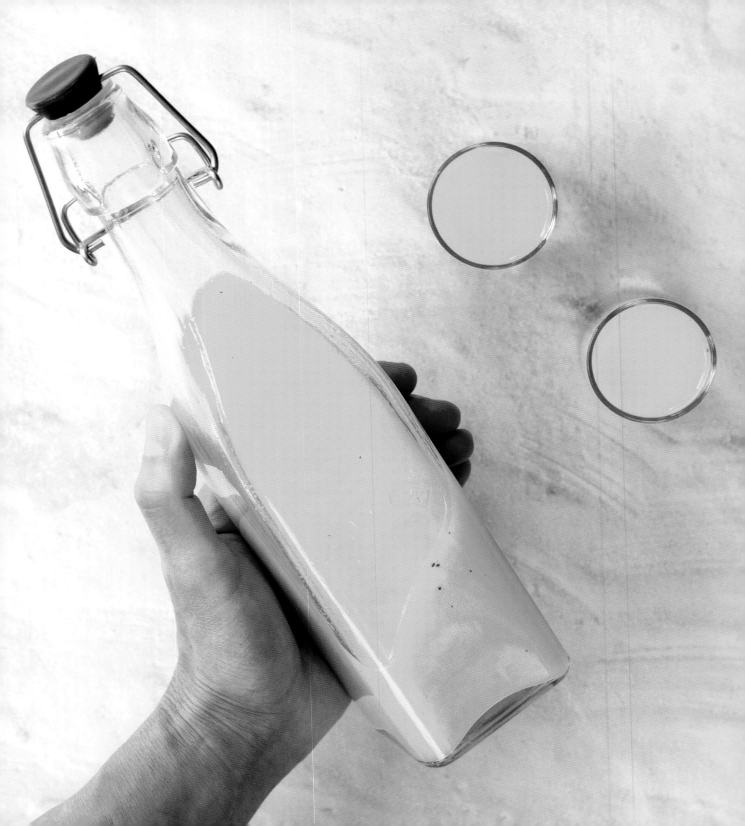

# wellness shot

Raw | anti-inflammatory | antibiotic  •  Yields: 6 servings

During the flu or cold season or when people around you tend to get sick, take extra precautions and add this shot to your morning routine. It is a dose of pure and potent nutrients straight from nature that will help you prevent and treat colds or the flu. If you are training hard and feeling a little run down, this is also an excellent natural anti-inflammatory remedy to help you with recovery. All you need is a juicer or blender and six ingredients. Cheers! To your health!

3 oranges, peeled

2 lemons, peeled

1 (1 to 2" [2.5- to 5-cm]) piece fresh ginger

1 (1" [2.5-cm]) piece fresh turmeric, or 1 tsp ground turmeric

10 to 12 drops culinary-grade oregano oil (depending on strength)

½ tsp freshly ground black pepper

### juicing method

Run the oranges, lemons, ginger and turmeric (if using fresh) through a juicer. Pour into a large glass jar with a lid. Add the oregano oil, ground turmeric powder (if using) and ground pepper. Close the jar tightly and shake well.

### blender method

In a blender, combine all the ingredients, except the oregano oil, and process until smooth.

Once blended, strain to remove the pulp.

Pour into a large glass jar with a lid. Add the oregano oil, close the jar tightly and shake well.

> **note:**
> This drink is quite intense, so if you can't handle the initial thought of drinking this in the morning, try biting into a fresh slice of orange or a piece of pineapple afterward.

## pro tips:

- Vitamins and minerals are generally best absorbed on an empty stomach, so we encourage you to drink your Wellness Shot first thing in the morning, before your first meal of the day.

- The best time to take a Wellness Shot is right when you're starting to feel a cold coming on, but honestly, having one of these once a day will keep you from getting sick in the first place. If you're already sick, try drinking two of these shots a day to help you get better faster.

# postrun juice

Raw | hydrating | mineral rich • Yields: 1 serving

Alkalizing and refreshing, this juice is a fantastic way to refuel and help speed up recovery after a long run or race. One of the great benefits of drinking fresh juice is that it floods your body with essential vitamins, minerals and proteins that can be absorbed within 15 to 20 minutes of consumption and without overloading digestion. Cucumber is cooling and thirst-quenching, and the highly superior water content helps regulate body temperature. Kale is packed with calcium and protein, which speeds up recovery and helps distribute nutrients through the body. Any juice that contains celery acts as the perfect postworkout tonic, as celery replaces lost electrolytes and rehydrates the body with its rich minerals. Finally, ginger and lemon are anti-inflammatory foods, very soothing to your joints.

1 large cucumber

Handful of kale

4 ribs celery

½ lemon, peeled

1 (1″ [2.5-cm]) piece fresh ginger

Cut the cucumber, kale and celery to fit through your juicer.

Juice all of the ingredients and enjoy right away.

**note:**

You can double this batch and keep extra in the fridge for when you crave a cold, uplifting midday snack.

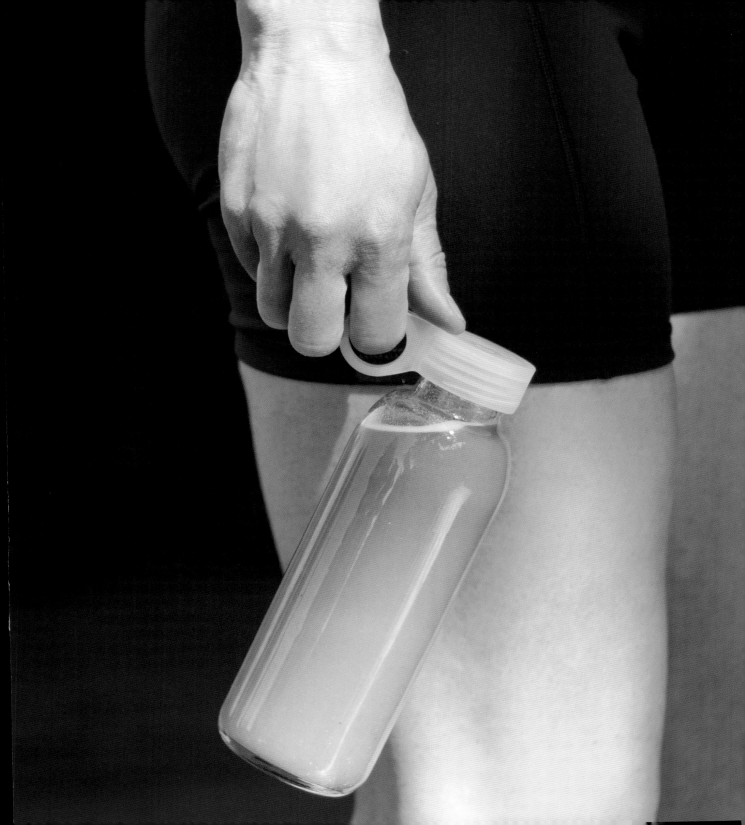

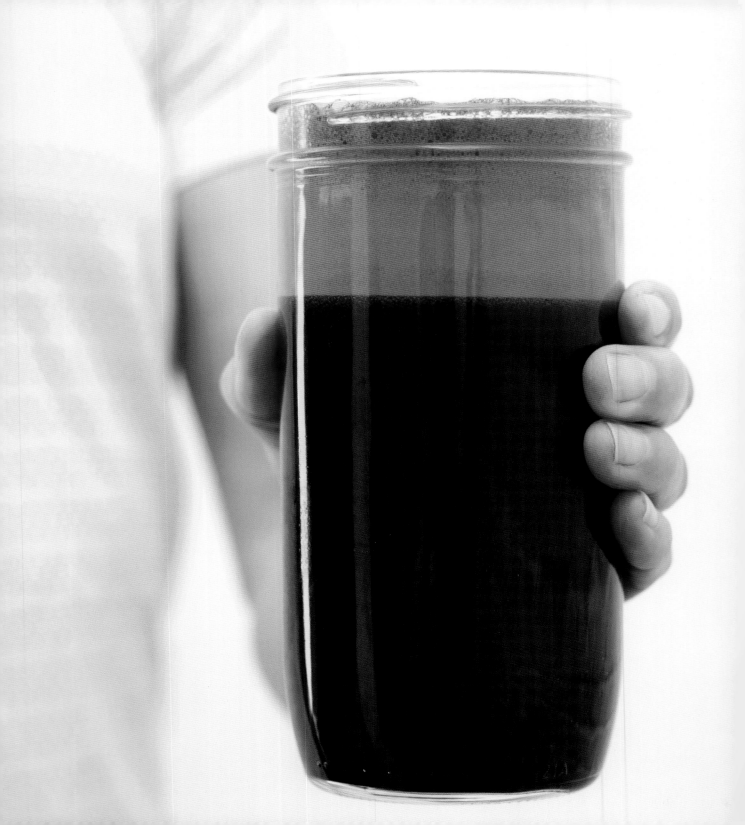

# blood transfusion juice

Raw | blood builder | detoxifying • Yields: 1 serving

The foundation of our health is based on the quality of our blood. This drink is a simple combination of four influential natural blood builders and cleansers, starting with beet juice—an incredible source of iron, folate and manganese and also one of the richest dietary sources of antioxidants and naturally occurring nitrates. Nitrates are compounds that improve blood flow throughout the body, including the brain, heart and muscles. Lemon acts as a blood purifier and cleansing agent. Another powerful addition is coconut water. One of the fascinating facts about coconut water is that it is incredibly similar to human plasma; it can be used in emergencies to rehydrate the human body if quickly administered intravenously. It's also used to improve blood circulation, lower elevated blood pressure, increase HDL (good) cholesterol and reduce the risk of heart attack and stroke. And last but certainly not least, this juice includes chlorella, extremely high in chlorophyll, which helps remove toxins from the blood and boost the immune system. Overall this health tonic is an excellent addition to your pre- and postworkout regimen!

1 young coconut, or 2 cups (475 ml) 100% coconut water

1 lemon, peeled

2 medium beets, peeled and cut into small pieces

2 tsp (4 g) chlorella

Crack open the young coconut (if using) and drain the coconut water into a blender container.

**using a juicer**
Run the lemon and beets through a juicer and add the juice to a blender with the coconut water and the chlorella powder. Gently blend on low speed for 5 seconds.

Drink immediately.

**without a juicer**
In a blender, combine all the ingredients, except the chlorella, and blend until smooth.

Using a fine-mesh metal strainer or a metal coffee filter, strain the juice into a large glass. Add the chlorella and stir.

**notes:**

- You can get 100% coconut water in many health food shops or could even buy a whole coconut and use the fresh coconut water, which of course is better as it is more whole.

- Beet juice can turn your urine and stools red—it's nothing to worry about!

- Beets contain oxalates; anyone with kidney problems should consult a doctor before consuming beet juice.

# raw power smoothie

Raw | meal replacement | muscle recovery  •  Yields: 1 serving

A high-quality, nutrient-dense, protein-packed, postworkout meal refuels your body and helps build lean muscle. On those days when your training session was extra intense, a liquid meal is the best option. Our go-to postworkout choice is this smoothie, which is easy to prepare and will leave you feeling energized, hydrated and ready to tackle the rest of your day.

1 cup (240 ml) purified water

1 orange, peeled and cut into chunks

1 fresh or frozen banana

1 cup (150 g) frozen berries (blueberries or raspberries are our favorite)

3 to 4 handfuls of leafy greens (spinach, kale, chard or romaine lettuce)

2 Medjool dates, pitted

2 tbsp (22 g) hemp hearts

1 tsp coconut butter, almond butter or tahini

1 tbsp (6 g) spirulina or chlorella powder

1 thumb-size piece fresh turmeric, or 1 tsp ground if fresh isn't available

Pinch of freshly ground black pepper

In a high-speed blender, combine all the ingredients and blend until smooth and creamy.

**note:**
Always strive to use fresh, raw, organic ingredients.

## pro tip:

To maximize the benefits from your training, drink this smoothie—or your interpretation of one like it—within 45 to 90 minutes after a workout.

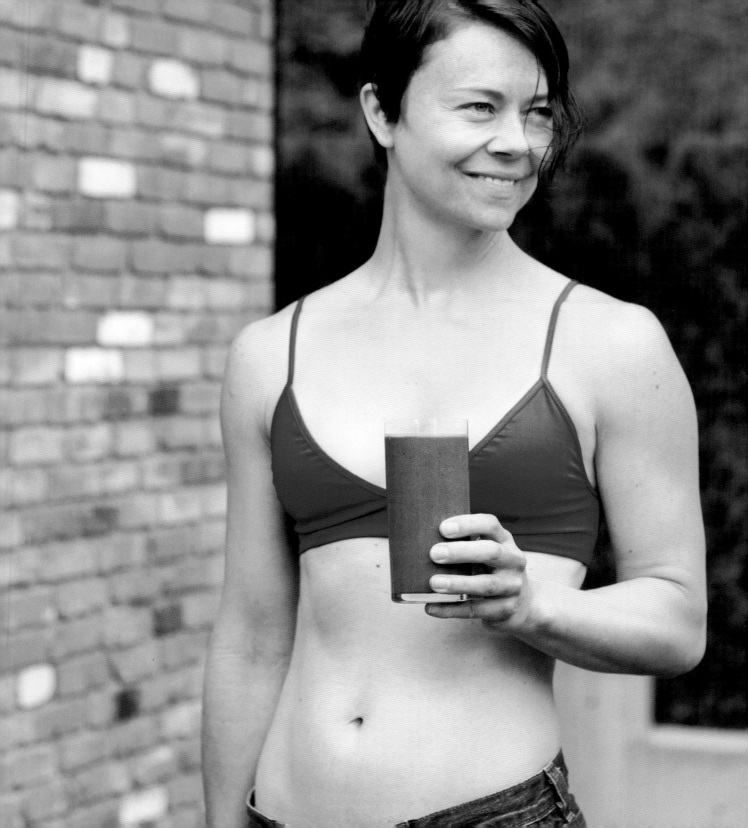

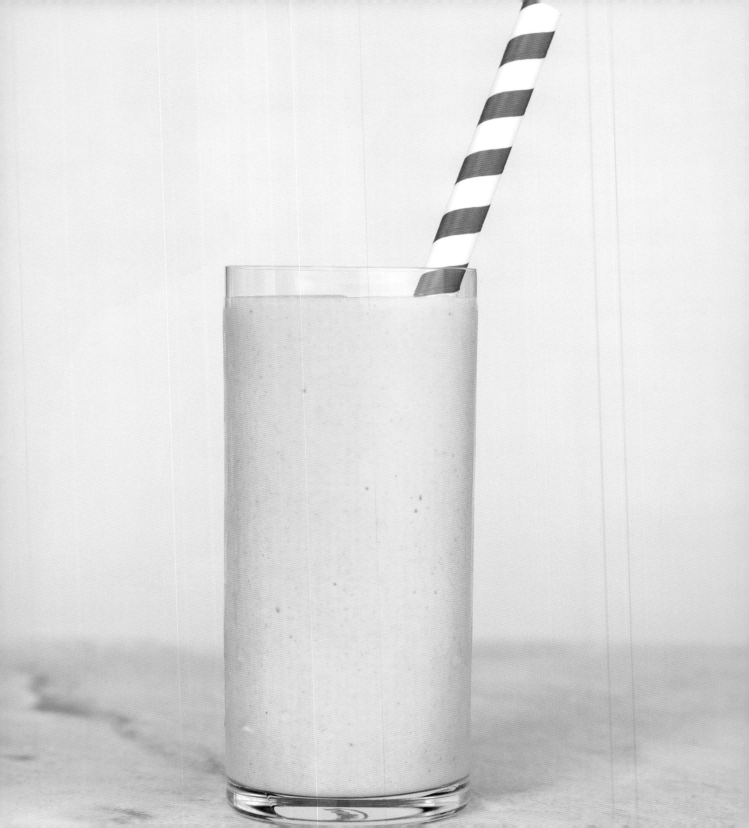

# golden colada recovery smoothie

Raw | anti-inflammatory | digestive aid • Yields: 1 serving

This recovery smoothie is a delicious way to feed your fatigued muscles after a strenuous endurance or a high-intensity workout. The golden color comes from turmeric, an anti-inflammatory powerhouse that will also reduce muscle and joint pain. Ginger and pineapple pack many antioxidants that are responsible for helping your body recover between workouts, plus they both contain enzymes that help with digestion and metabolism of food. It's one of our ultimate go-to postworkout smoothies.

1 (1" [2.5-cm]) piece fresh turmeric, peeled, or 1 tsp ground turmeric

1 (1" [2.5-cm]) piece fresh ginger, peeled

1 frozen banana

1 cup (165 g) fresh pineapple chunks

1 cup (240 ml) plant-based mylk (pages 50–53)

1 tbsp (11 g) hemp hearts

Juice of 1 small lime

In a blender, combine all the ingredients and blend until smooth and creamy.

Drink right away.

note:

Try to drink your smoothie right away. After 15 minutes, light and air will destroy much of the nutrients. If you can't drink it fresh, transfer it to an airtight dark glass container until you're ready.

# maca-mint smoothie

Raw | energy & endurance | preworkout • Yields: 1 serving

A smoothie is a perfect preworkout liquid "meal" that can easily be customized depending on your hunger level and your workout goals. This smoothie is full of whole foods, including a sneaky serving of spinach! The simple carbohydrates from the bananas will provide your muscles with easy-to-digest preworkout fuel to sustain your energy throughout demanding training sessions, and the maca powder will help increase energy, stamina and endurance.

2 tbsp (18 g) raw cashews

1 heaping handful of baby spinach

1 cup (240 ml) almond mylk (page 50)

2 frozen bananas, chopped

1 tbsp (15 ml) fresh lemon juice

20 fresh mint leaves

1 tsp maca powder

1 tbsp (8 g) cacao nibs (optional)

In a high-speed blender, combine all the ingredients, except the cacao nibs, and blend until smooth and creamy.

Top with the cacao nibs, if you like.

Enjoy 60 to 90 minutes before training.

# watermelon rehydrator

Raw | hydrating | natural electrolytes • Yields: 24 oz (710 ml); 1 or 2 servings

Friends, this recipe is a game changer and has been an enormous help in our workout recovery. Made from only a few simple ingredients, this is the perfect way to stay hydrated during your rides and runs but also a super-refreshing postworkout recovery drink. It contains natural functional nutrients, including electrolytes, potassium and L-citrulline—an amino acid that helps relieve muscle soreness after an intense exercise.

3 cups (450 g) chopped watermelon, preferably with seeds

1 cup (240 ml) purified water

Juice of ½ lemon

1 tsp kelp flakes, or pinch of Celtic sea salt

In a blender, combine all the ingredients. Blend until liquefied. Pour into a glass bottle with a lid or a sports bottle. Chill until you're ready to serve, or drink it right away.

*See image on page 94.

## pro tip:

If your workout is on the more intense side and longer than 75 to 90 minutes, add 1 tablespoon (15 ml) of a natural sweetener, such as raw agave nectar or maple syrup, to the mixture.

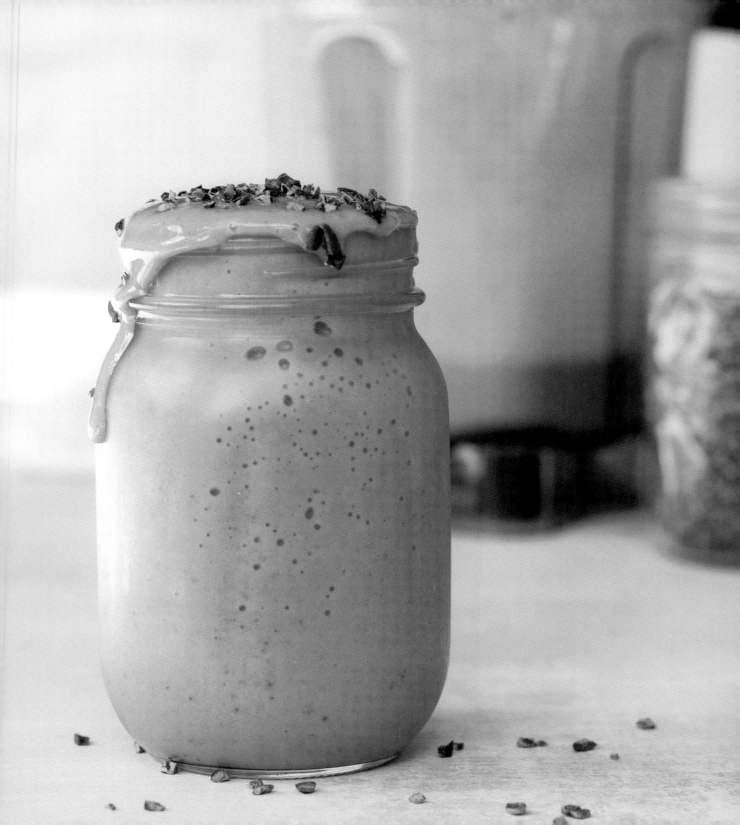

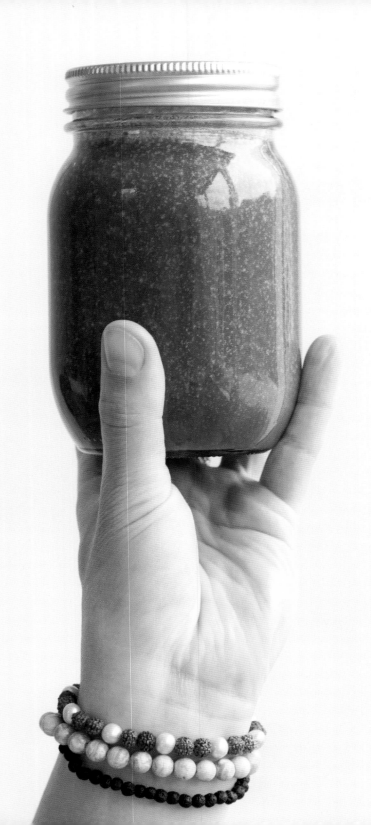

# plant-powered muscle mylk

Raw | protein rich | recovery fuel  •  Yields: 1 serving

Are you looking for a way to refuel your body after a workout? Look no further—this muscle mylk was created with one main goal in mind: to replenish. Whether you are refueling after an intense workout session or looking for a meal that will supply you with nutritious energy to last you for hours, this green "mylkshake" will do the trick! It's a two-part drink—one part coconut milk and the other part green vegetables and fruit juice. It may seem weird, but trust us, it's delicious! Overall, this is a highly nutritious liquid meal that will supply a healthy dose of plant-based protein and rehydrate your body with electrolytes lost during exercise.

5 ribs celery

1 bunch kale

½ bunch cilantro

2 green apples

1 young coconut, or 1 cup (240 ml) nut mylk (coconut or almond mylk, page 50)

1 Medjool date, pitted

Run the celery, kale, cilantro and apples through a juicer. Set aside.

If using a fresh coconut, crack it open. Empty the coconut water through a fine-mesh strainer into a bowl. Scoop the meat out of the coconut, using a large spoon.

In a blender, combine the coconut meat and water (or nut mylk, if using) with the date and blast on high speed for 30 to 60 seconds, or until smooth and creamy.

Add the green juice to the blender and blend well until all the ingredients are combined, about 30 seconds. Serve immediately.

**note:**

This highly nutritious and vibrant green drink was inspired by Lou Corona and Dan McDonald. Thank you, gentlemen, for sharing your knowledge and experience of raw food living. You rock!

**pro tips:**

- Serve over ice, if desired.
- Lou's Tip: If you do not have a juicer, it is okay to use a blender, though you may have to add purified water to get the mixture to blend. If you use a blender, pour the juice through a nut milk bag or fine strainer set over a bowl.

# chocolate muscle mylk

*Raw | strengthens endurance | hormone balancing*  •  Yields: 1 serving

Okay, I admit it. I consumed a fair amount of "muscle milk" protein drinks in my early 20s. You know, those ready-to-drink shakes that claim to make you stronger, leaner, faster? The trouble is that with a whopping 40 ingredients on the label, they're a far cry from healthy food! This new and improved version of muscle milk will give you power and strength. It packs healthy and easily digestible protein, carbs and fat. This drink is soothing and healing for you, especially after a hike or workout session. And the best part is, it will help you build and maintain muscle mass as you transition to a plant-based diet. It tastes great and is supereasy to make.

1½ cups (355 ml) almond mylk (page 50)

1 tbsp (7 g) raw cacao powder

2 Medjool dates, pitted

1 tsp maca powder

2 Brazil nuts

Pinch of sea salt

In a high-speed blender, combine all the ingredients and blend until smooth and creamy.

**note:**

You can double this batch and keep extra in the fridge for when you crave a cold, uplifting midday snack.

## pro tip:

If you're sensitive to caffeine or struggling with adrenal fatigue, consider replacing the cacao with carob powder. Unlike chocolate, carob does not contain any stimulative alkaloids and won't overstimulate your central nervous system.

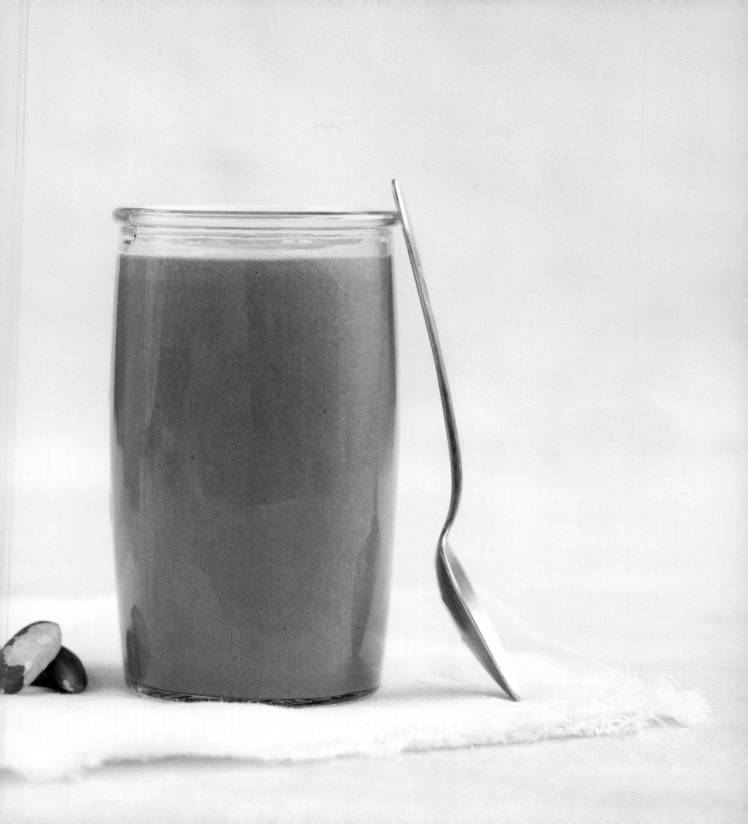

# ginger ale workout tonic

Raw | energy boost | preworkout fuel  •  Yields: 1 serving

This upgraded version of ginger ale is best consumed before and during a longer or more intense workout. Ginger is a high-alkaline rhizome that can help control lactic acid buildup. When you're pushing through reps, lactic acid buildup causes that burning feeling in your muscles, which can keep you from doing extra sets. The pineapple is high in a digestive enzyme called bromelain, supporting easy digestion and therefore reducing the risk of stomach cramps or side stitches. Overall this tonic will provide your muscles with easy-to-digest preworkout fuel and naturally boost your overall athletic performance.

1 (1″ [2.5-cm]) piece fresh ginger, peeled

1 cup (155 g) chopped fresh pineapple

1 lemon, peeled

1 lime, peeled

1 tbsp (15 ml) raw agave nectar

1 cup (240 ml) mineral water or coconut water

1 cup (240 ml) purified water, if using a blender

### juicing method
Run the ginger, pineapple, lemon and lime through a juicer.

Pour the juice into a large glass and mix in the agave and mineral water. Stir and enjoy 20 to 30 minutes before a training session.

### blender method
In a blender, combine the ginger, pineapple, lemon and lime, add the purified water and blend thoroughly until the texture is smooth. Strain the juice through a strainer and discard the pulp.

Pour the strained juice into a large glass and mix in the agave and mineral water. Stir and enjoy 20 to 30 minutes before a training session.

### pro tip:
You can add another tablespoon (15 ml) of raw agave if you are planning a workout that will exceed 3 hours.

# sleep tonic

Immunity boosting | antistress | sleep promoting  •  Yields: 1 serving

Sleep is an integral part of recovery—your body regenerates muscle cells during sleep by releasing growth hormone. If your stress levels are too high, your body will not be able to get into a deep phase of sleep, and your recovery, as well as performance, will suffer. This sleep-promoting tonic made with ashwagandha is an old Ayurvedic remedy traditionally taken before bed to promote restful sleep. Ashwagandha is a powerful adaptogenic herb, meaning it helps the body restore its balance. It does this by assisting the body in regulating its response to both internal and external stressors, such as anxiety and environmental toxins, while strengthening the immune system, controlling blood sugar and toning the adrenals. Another fantastic benefit of ashwagandha is its unique ability to both energize and invigorate, and calm and relax—making this sleep tonic an excellent choice for those who have a difficult time getting going in the morning or falling asleep at night.

1 cup (240 ml) plant-based mylk (almond, coconut, quinoa, hemp, etc., pages 50–53)

½ tsp ground ashwagandha powder

½ tsp ground cinnamon, plus more for sprinkling

¼ tsp ground cardamom

1 tsp coconut oil

1 tbsp (15 ml) Date Syrup (page 56)

In a small pot, bring the mylk to a low simmer, but don't let it boil.

Meanwhile, in a blender, combine the ashwagandha, cinnamon, cardamom, coconut oil and date syrup.

Add the warm mylk and blend until smooth and creamy.

To serve, sprinkle ground cinnamon on top. Enjoy warm.

### a word of caution:

Ashwagandha is safe for most people to consume, but it may interact with thyroid, blood pressure and blood sugar medications. Pregnant and breastfeeding women, as well as people with autoimmune disorders such as rheumatoid arthritis or lupus, may need to avoid ashwagandha. Ashwagandha should not be taken with alcohol, sedatives or anxiolytics.

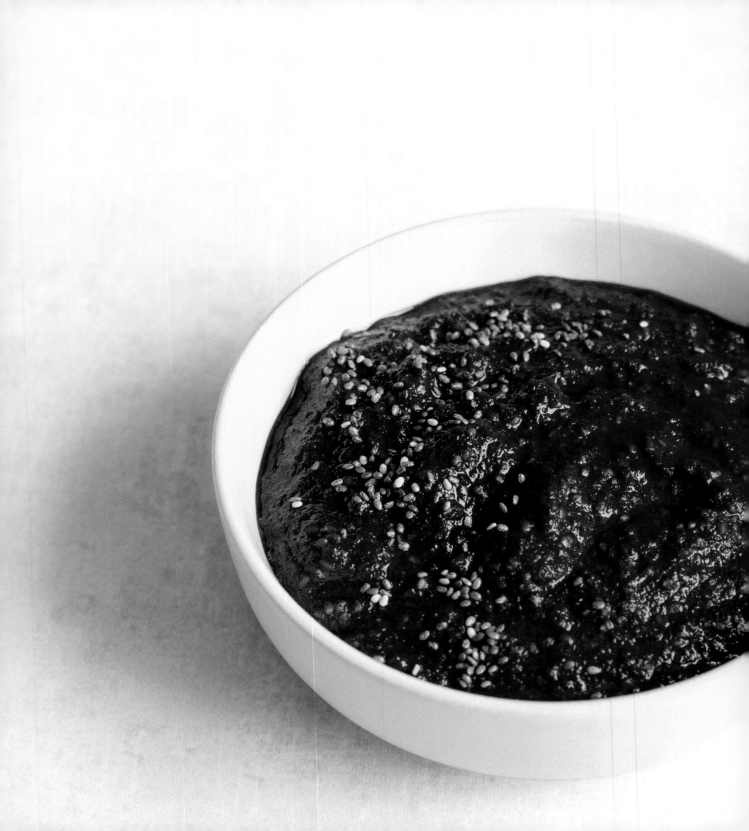

# berry chia energy gel

Raw | anti-inflammatory | improved performance  •  Yields: 3 or 4 servings

This gel is packed full of energizing nutrients that provide easily digestible nourishment for your long and intense workouts. Known as the "running food," chia seeds are a fantastic high-energy endurance food that dates as far back as the ancient Aztecs. Soldiers used to eat a daily serving of these tiny seeds to give them energy for running long distances and to sustain them for long periods of heat and thirst. When you pair chia seeds with natural sugar and electrolytes (as in this recipe), it creates the perfect fuel for before, during and after any high-intensity and endurance activities.

1 small beet, peeled and chopped

1 cup (150 g) fresh or frozen blueberries

1 tbsp (15 ml) fresh lime juice

1 tbsp (15 ml) raw agave nectar

¼ tsp ground turmeric

Pinch of sea salt

2 tbsp (20 g) chia seeds

In a blender or food processor, combine all the ingredients, except the chia seeds; process until the mixture reaches a smooth consistency. Transfer to a bowl and mix in the chia seeds. Cover the bowl with a plate or lid and refrigerate for at least 20 minutes.

When ready to use, divide the gel into small ziplock plastic bags or reusable gel containers.

This gel will keep for up to 3 days in the refrigerator, but it is best when consumed fresh.

## pro tip:

This gel is suggested for moderate-intensity activity that lasts up to 3 hours.

# salted caramel endurance gel

Raw | sustained energy | stomach soothing   •   Soaking time: 5 to 10 minutes | Yields: 2 servings

If you enjoy endurance sports or long outdoor adventures, you will appreciate this recipe. I started experimenting with making my own gels during my first ultramarathon training. I wanted something to take with me for the long runs that would give me quick energy when needed without upsetting my stomach. This gel was a real winner. It's tasty, and unlike most commercial products, it doesn't contain any artificial flavors or colors, only natural living ingredients to fuel your next big adventure.

2 Medjool dates, pitted

2 tbsp (32 g) raw nut butter

1 tsp maca powder

¼ cup (60 ml) agave nectar

½ tsp sea salt

1 (½" [1.3-cm]) piece fresh ginger, grated

¼ tsp ground cardamom (optional)

Soak the dates in water for 5 to 10 minutes, then drain.

In a high-speed blender or food processor, combine the soaked dates with all the other ingredients and blend until smooth.

Divide the energy gel between 2 (3-ounce [90-ml]) GoToobs.

Consume the gels during your workout. Six ounces (180 ml) was more than enough for a 3-hour run.

## pro tip:

This gel will provide balanced, slow-burning energy—great fuel for endurance athletes who are on the road for the long haul, be it on an ultramarathon, a long hike, a long ride or any other adventure.

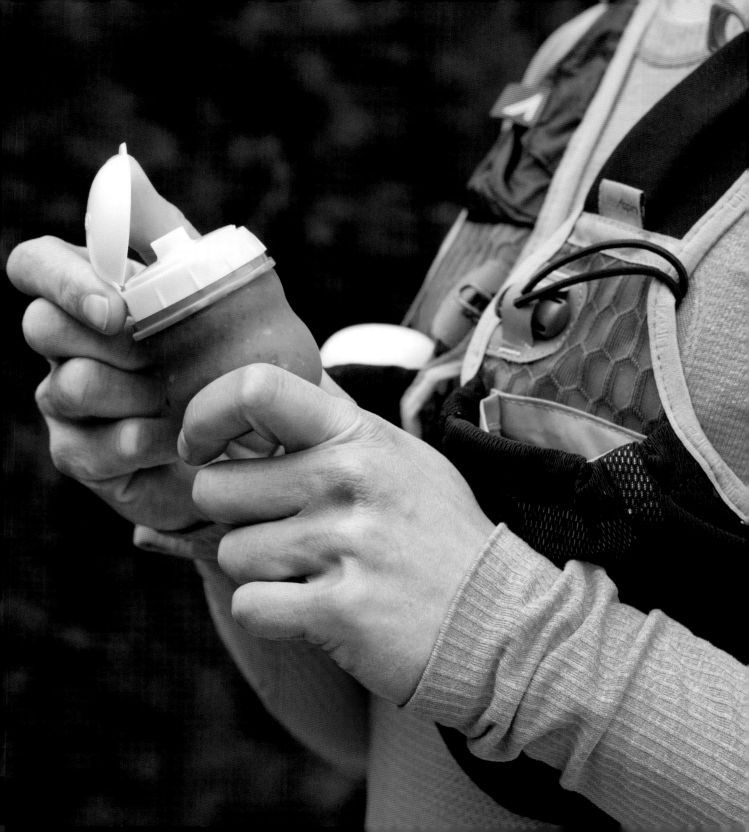

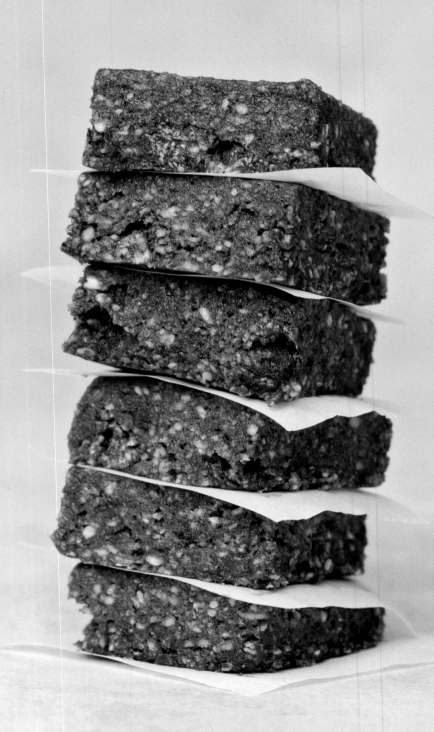

# spirulina-golden berry power bars

Raw | high-energy | prevents fatigue • Yields: 8 bars

Let's face it—energy bars are here to stay. They are convenient fuel for anyone active, athletic, or who lives a busy life but wants to eat healthy when away from home or after workouts. This bar is a perfect example of a high-quality, plant-powered snack that will satisfy your cravings between meals. It has a 60 percent healthy saturated fat ratio and is packed full of antioxidants. It doesn't contain any nuts, but has a full protein profile with seeds and spirulina, providing you with the amino acid building blocks that you need for optimal recovery, plus antioxidants-rich golden berries to help reduce the inflammatory response caused by exercise.

1 cup (145 g) mixed raw seeds (pumpkin, sunflower, sesame, hemp)

1 tbsp (10 g) chia seeds

1 cup (178 g) Medjool dates (about 10 large), pitted

2 tbsp (3 g) chopped fresh mint

2 tsp (4 g) spirulina powder

1 tbsp (15 ml) fresh lime juice

½ cup (112 g) golden berries

In a food processor fitted with the S blade, combine all the ingredients, except the golden berries.

Process until a coarse dough has formed (this may take a couple of minutes). Stop the machine and check the consistency—pinch the dough between 2 fingers and make sure it sticks together easily so that your bars don't end up crumbly. If the dough is too dry, add a small amount of water—about ½ teaspoon at a time—and blend again until the desired stickiness is achieved.

Add the golden berries and pulse several times until they're just coarsely chopped, to give the bars a nice texture.

Place a large sheet of parchment paper on a flat surface and tip out the dough on top. Gather into a solid mass in the center, then fold the parchment paper over the top and, using a rolling pin, roll flat until about ¼ inch (6 mm) thick.

Place in the freezer for a few hours, then carefully use a knife or cookie cutter to cut the bars into your desired shapes.

Store in an airtight glass container for 2 to 3 weeks or in the freezer for up to 3 months.

**note:**

If the dates are really hard and dry, rehydrate them for about 15 minutes in enough warm water to cover them. Be sure to drain the excess water before adding the dates to the recipe.

**pro tip:**

Golden berries, a.k.a. gooseberries or Incan berries, are an amazing source of vitamin C, antioxidants and protein, just to name a few of their nutritional benefits. They are worth including in your diet; however, if you cannot find them, you could replace them with cranberries or raisins.

# coco-mango performance bars

Raw | sustained energy | anti-inflammatory   •   Yields: 6 bars

In our "grab and go" world, sometimes we need a little help filling in the nutritional gap, and energy bars are a convenient way to satisfy those needs. Unfortunately, most store-bought bars today have a long list of ingredients, few of which sound like real food. We encourage you to start making your energy snacks instead. You won't find any unnecessary added junk in these bars—just good, whole ingredients with an awesome taste and burst of energy. They contain 9 grams of easily digestible protein and a healthy dose of fiber that will help you maintain energy throughout the day or during a long-lasting training session.

1 cup (178 g) soft Medjool dates (about 10), pitted

1 cup (85 g) shredded unsweetened coconut

½ cup (68 g) raw macadamia nuts or cashews

¼ cup (41 g) fresh or frozen mango

1 tbsp (10 g) chia seeds

2 tsp (10 g) maca powder

2 tbsp (15 g) cacao nibs

2 tbsp (18 g) raw nuts/seeds (your favorite kind)

In a food processor, grind together all the ingredients, except the 2 tablespoons (18 g) of nuts/seeds, until a coarse dough has formed (this process may take a couple of minutes).

Stop the machine and check the consistency—pinch the dough between 2 fingers and make sure it sticks together easily, so that your bars don't end up crumbly. If the dough is too dry, add a small amount of water—about ½ teaspoon at a time—and blend again until your desired stickiness is achieved. Then, add the 2 tablespoons (18 g) of nuts/seeds and pulse several times until coarsely chopped, to give the bars a nice texture.

To shape into bars: Turn out the mixture onto a clean work surface. Flatten with your hands. Place a sheet of parchment paper on top, then roll out with a rolling pin to your desired thickness. Cut into bars.

Alternatively, form the mixture into a brick, then cut into slices. Or press the mixture into a parchment paper–lined baking dish or brownie pan, refrigerate for about 5 hours, then slice into bars.

As the bars dry in the fridge, they become easier to handle and slice.

Store in an airtight glass container for 1 week or in the freezer for up to 1 month.

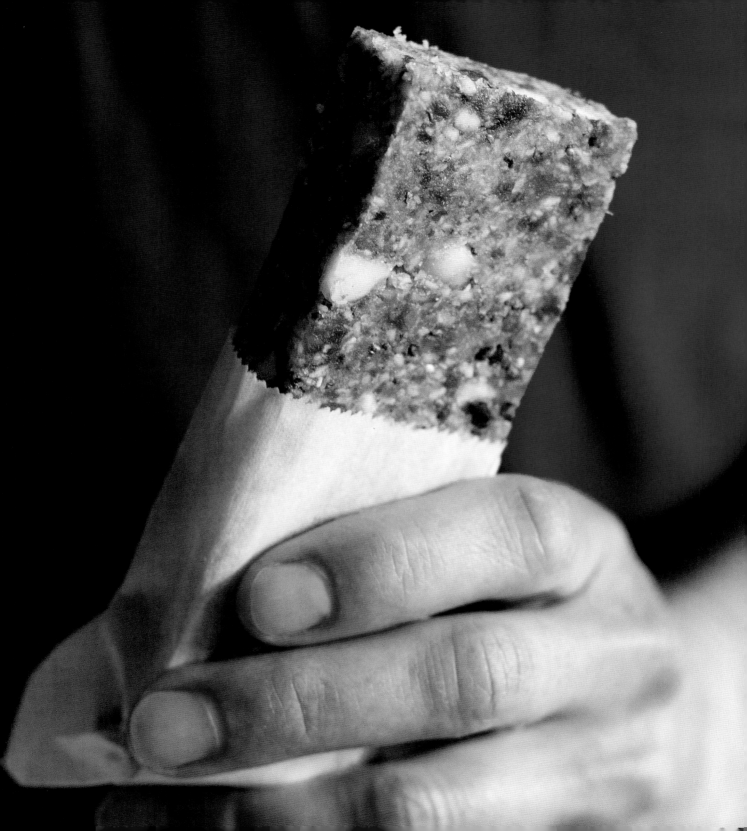

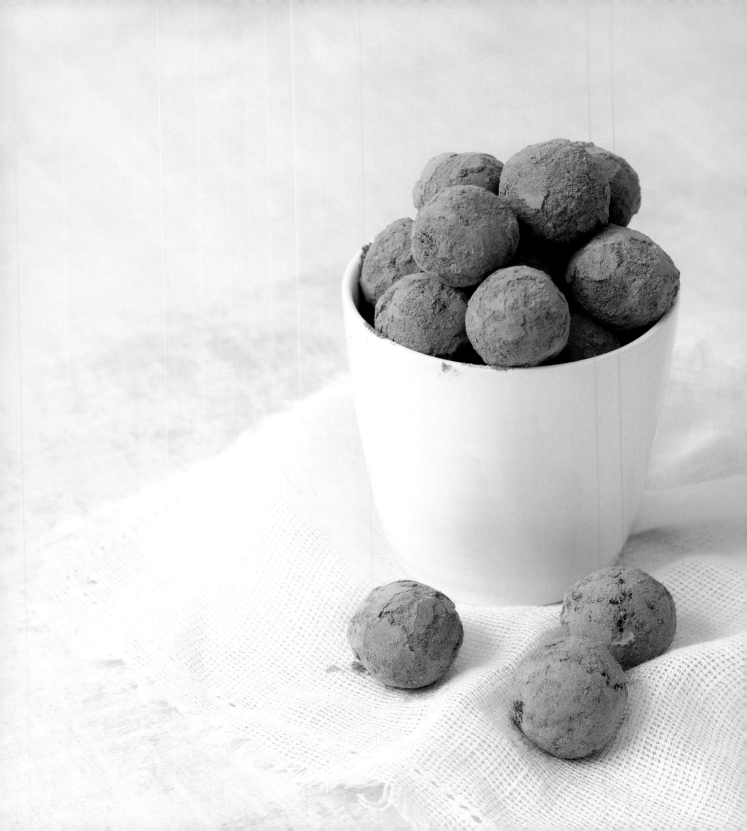

# popeye protein balls

Raw | bone strengthening | workout fuel  •  Soaking time: 15 minutes | Yields: 20 to 26 balls

Popeye was right about spinach helping you grow strong muscles—rich in calcium, magnesium and iron, spinach also contains natural chemicals that help build muscles by speeding up the body's conversion of protein into muscle mass. In honor of our childhood superhero, these protein balls include a healthy dose of spinach. Don't worry, you won't taste the spinach, but it's there, and it adds proper nutrition. Whether at work, after lunch, as a preworkout snack or a postworkout protein, these superfood-packed balls are a wholesome but delicious choice!

1 cup (125 g) raw hazelnuts

¼ cup (35 g) pumpkin seeds

Handful of fresh baby spinach

2 tbsp (14 g) raw cacao or carob powder

1 cup (145 g) raisins, soaked in water for 15 minutes, rinsed and drained

2 tbsp (15 g) hemp protein powder

1 tsp ground cinnamon

Pinch of Himalayan pink salt

2 to 4 tbsp (30 to 60 g) superfood powder (açai, maqui, maca, spirulina, matcha or moringa), depending on potency, for dusting (optional)

In a food processor fitted with the S blade, combine all the ingredients, except the superfood powder, and process until the mixture forms a ball. Do not overprocess! If you do, the dough will become too soft. (If that happens, add up to 2 tablespoons [18 g] of pumpkin seeds and refrigerate for 30 minutes before forming into balls.)

To shape into balls, use a tablespoon or your hands to scoop the mixture (however much you like to make 1 ball) and roll between the palms of your hands.

Place on a plate and refrigerate for a minimum of 1 hour before serving.

If desired, before refrigerating, roll the balls in a plate of superfood powder to dust their exterior.

**note:**

If you have the time, we highly suggest you presoak the hazelnuts before using. See page 28 for details.

# epic power orbs

On-the-go snack | protein rich | energy boost  •  Yields: 20 to 26 orbs

Whether you are trying to fit a snack in around your next meeting, school run, gym session or marathon, these superfoods and nutritionally balanced orbs are an excellent choice. Made with energy-packed apricots and figs as well as protein-rich nuts and goji berries, they are the perfect combination to help improve your performance and support recovery. The best thing is that you can make a big batch and they seem to keep forever in the fridge in an airtight container.

½ cup (65 g) dried apricots

½ cup (75 g) dried figs

1½ cups (128 g) shredded unsweetened coconut

½ cup (70 g) raw cashews

½ cup (50 g) walnuts

¼ cup (25 g) goji berries

¼ cup (60 ml) fresh orange juice

½ tsp ground cardamom

Pinch of sea salt

Soak the apricots and figs in warm water for 15 to 20 minutes. Drain and rinse.

In a food processor fitted with the S blade, combine all the ingredients, including the apricots and figs. Using the pulse button, process until chopped. Check the seasoning and adjust as necessary.

With an ice-cream scoop or melon baller, form balls 1 inch (2.5 cm) in diameter. You can also roll scoops of the dough between the palms of your hands to form balls.

### baked
Preheat the oven to 300°F (150°C). Line a baking sheet with parchment paper.

Place the orbs on the prepared baking sheet.

Bake for around 25 minutes, or until just starting to brown around the edges.

### dehydrated
Place the orbs on a mesh or nonstick sheet on a dehydrator tray and dry at 115°F (46°C) for 12 hours, turning over after 6 hours. Alternatively, dry in an oven heated to its lowest setting.

Remove from the oven or dehydrator and store in a sealed jar for up to 10 days.

note:

If you have the time, we highly suggest you presoak the nuts before using. See page 28 for details.

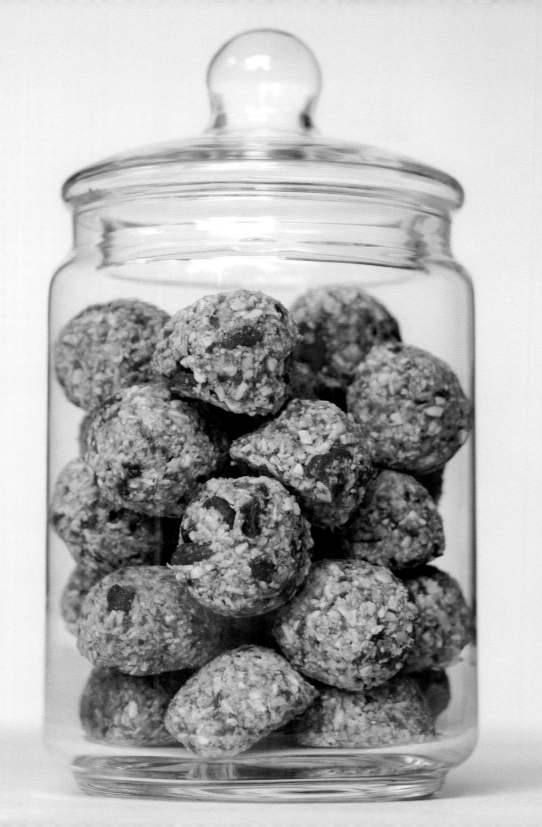

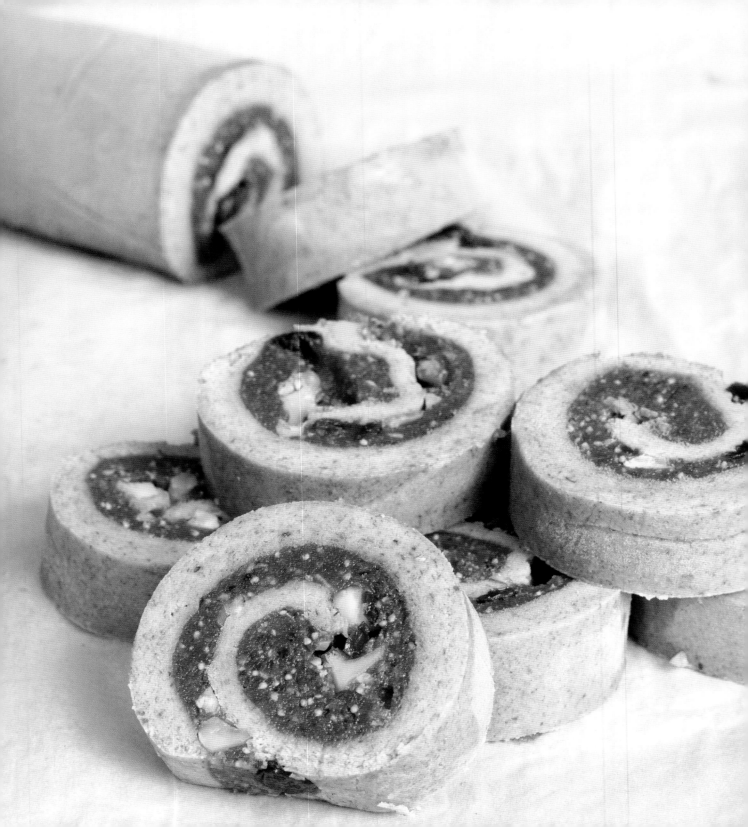

# raw cinnamon rolls

Raw | bone strengthening | midworkout fuel  •  Yields: 12 rolls

Here is a cinnamon roll you can feel great about—an excellent clean and tasty bite-sized snack that delivers on all the essential needs for any athlete. The combination of raw agave and sun-dried figs will provide you with the sustainable, balanced release of energy for best performance—without a spike and crash. We like to use these rolls as a midride/-run/-hike fuel source. It's always great to reach into the back pocket of your jersey or backpack and refuel with a tasty snack!

## dough

½ cup (84 g) flaxseeds

1 cup (145 g) almonds or (100 g) pecans

¼ cup (60 ml) raw agave nectar

## filling

1 cup (150 g) dried figs, stemmed and diced (about 10 figs)

¼ cup (60 ml) water

2 tbsp (15 g) ground cinnamon

¾ tsp ground cardamom

¼ tsp sea salt

2 tbsp (18 g) raisins (optional)

2 tbsp (13 g) chopped pecans or walnuts (optional)

Prepare the dough: In a coffee or spice grinder, grind the flaxseeds to a fine powder. Transfer to a food processor and blend with the almonds until a flourlike consistency is formed.

Add the agave and process into a workable dough, adding a touch of water, if needed. Remove the dough and place between 2 large sheets of parchment paper. Using a rolling pin or your hands, flatten into a large square. Peel off the top layer of paper and set the dough aside.

Prepare the filling: In a clean food processor, puree the figs, water, cinnamon, cardamom and salt into a thick paste. Spread the mixture evenly over your dough and sprinkle with raisins and chopped nuts, if desired.

Next, roll the dough into a tight cylinder, as if you were making sushi, using the parchment paper as the mat. Place your roll in the freezer to set for about half an hour, then remove and cut into 12 equal pieces.

Store the rolls in a glass container in the freezer. They will keep for up to 2 weeks.

### pro tip:

When selecting an agave nectar, look for one that is both raw and organic.

# endurance snack mix

Raw | iron rich | muscle & bone builder • Yields: 3 cups (365 g)

This mix is probably one of the most accessible snacks to throw together. Nuts, seeds and naturally dried fruits are high-energy food that can provide you with fuel for long, intense workouts. The inclusion of seaweed in this mix is a nutritious way to increase the mineral content in your diet and replenish electrolytes lost during physical activity. So, whether you are hiking, biking, driving your kids around town or playing, this mix offers a sustainable energy boost to charge you up throughout the day.

½ cup (62 g) raw pistachios

1 cup (140 g) raw pumpkin seeds

½ cup (43 g) unsweetened large coconut flakes

¼ cup (35 g) raisins

¼ cup (25 g) goji berries

½ cup (56 g) dried mulberries

Handful of dried dulse, or 1 sheet nori, cut into bite-sized pieces

In a medium-sized bowl, combine all the ingredients and toss well.

Portion into several servings in either snack-sized paper bags, reusable bags or small glass jars. You can then keep them in your backpack, purse, gym bag, car or any other place that's convenient.

They will keep for several weeks in the fridge or freezer.

### note:

Choose raw, unsalted and sulfite-free ingredients. Look to buy in bulk as well (see resources section on page 216), as this can be more cost effective and environmentally friendly.

### pro tip:

Keep it interesting week after week by creating your own combinations and mixing a variety of raw nuts, seeds, sun-dried fruits and sea vegetables.

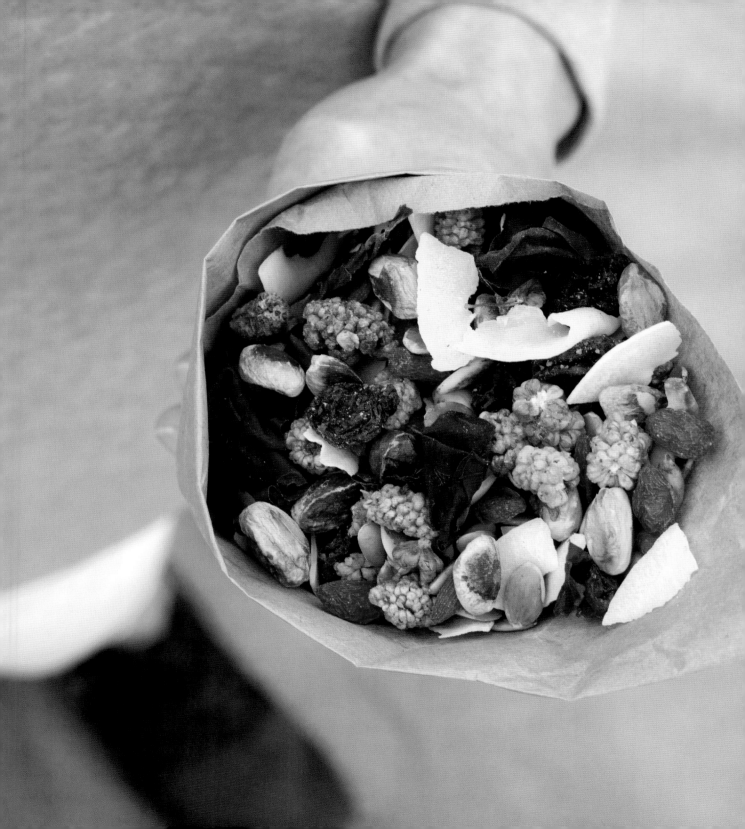

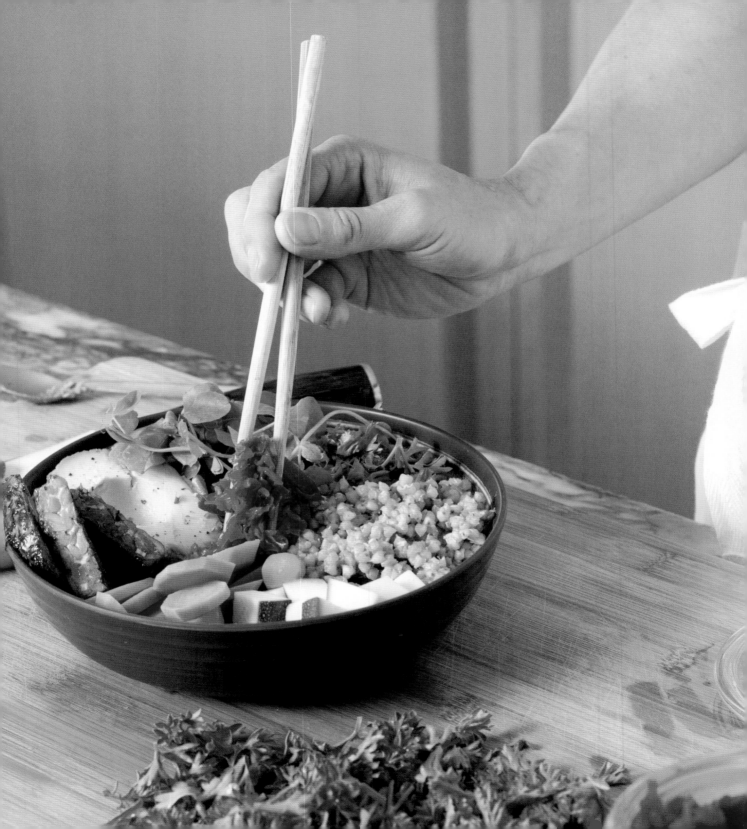

# power
## main meals

We often get asked by friends and family to create healthy versions of their favorite comfort meals, and we love this challenge! It's our mission to show you that just because you're eating healthy doesn't mean you have to give up great-tasting food. You will find a comforting tortilla soup (page 136) that takes less than ten minutes to make, a step-by-step process on how to build your own Nourish Bowl (page 146), a crowd-pleasing burger (page 157) and more. These delicious, satisfying and family-friendly meals are made with love and layered with flavor. Give these recipes a try; we are confident you will enjoy the results, both at the dinner table and during your performance.

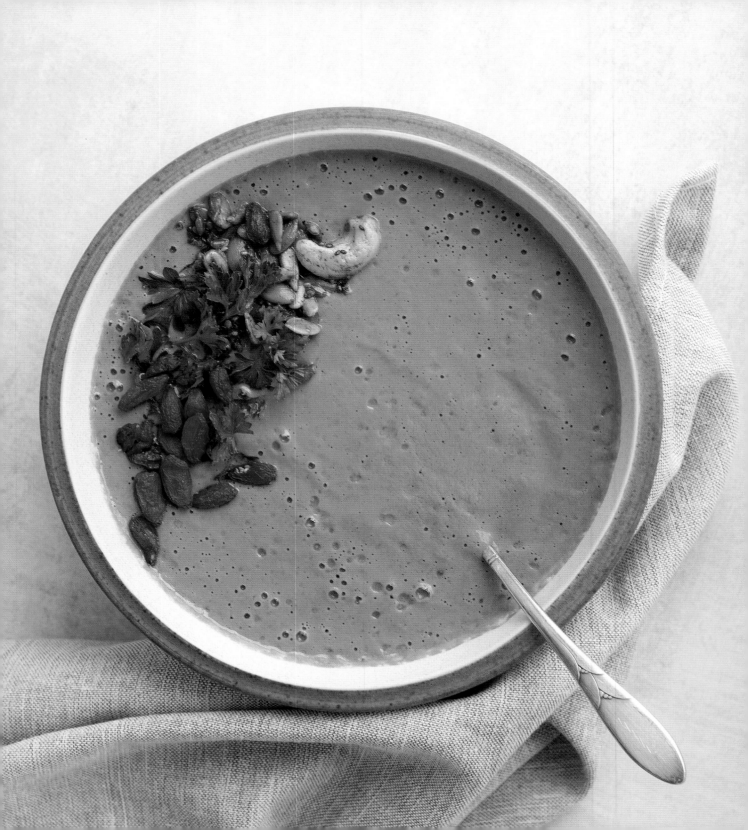

# green goddess soup

Raw | protein and mineral rich  •  Soaking time: 8 hours or overnight | Yields: 2 servings

This smooth and creamy soup makes an appearance for dinner in our house at least once per week. It's packed full of iron from both the greens and the pumpkin seeds. The addition of fresh lemon juice not only balances the flavor of this nutritious soup, but also helps increase the iron absorption from plant-based foods.

¼ cup (35 g) raw pumpkin seeds, soaked in water for 8 hours or overnight

2 tbsp (16 g) sesame seeds, soaked in water for 8 hours or overnight

3 cups (90 g) fresh spinach

1 cup (60 g) fresh parsley, chopped

Juice of 1 lemon

2 cups (475 ml) purified water

2 Medjool dates, pitted

1 tsp sea salt

½ tsp freshly ground black pepper

1 small clove garlic, peeled

½ tsp fennel seeds (optional)

**to serve**

Chopped fresh herbs

Superfood Salad Topper (page 60; optional)

In a high-speed or regular blender (see pro tip), combine all the ingredients and blend thoroughly until the texture is smooth and creamy.

If you used a regular blender, you may pour the mixture into a saucepan and gently warm over low heat, stirring and watching carefully so as not to overheat it. It should be warm enough to enjoy but not too hot as the heat would damage the precious vitamins and enzymes that make it so nourishing.

To serve, garnish the soup with chopped herbs and sprinkle with a spoonful of Superfood Salad Topper, if desired.

## pro tip:

Blending raw soups in a high-speed blender, such as Vitamix, will warm the liquids gently. This will ensure that you are not damaging these heat-sensitive essential nutrients, such as vitamins, minerals and enzymes, which would normally not survive the traditional cooking methods. Plus, you can have an amazing nutrient-dense meal ready to enjoy in less than 10 minutes!

# warming tortilla soup

Raw | nutrient dense | high fiber  •  Yields: 2 servings

A low-fat yet hearty and delicious raw-style tortilla soup blended with fresh and sun-dried tomatoes, bell peppers, celery, fresh cilantro, a splash of citrus, warming spices . . . and let's not forget that avocado that gives this soup its creamy texture. This soup would be perfect any time of the day—enjoy it chilled during the summer months, or warm it up a bit for those chillier days or when you crave a comfort food at the end of a busy day.

¼ cup (28 g) sun-dried tomatoes

3 tomatoes, coarsely chopped

2 large red, orange or yellow bell peppers (or a combination), seeded and coarsely chopped

2 large ribs celery, coarsely chopped

½ packed cup (20 g) fresh cilantro

½ cup (120 ml) purified water

1 tbsp (15 ml) fresh lime juice

1 date, pitted

1 tsp sea salt

1 tsp ground coriander

½ tsp smoked paprika

1 to 3 cloves garlic (depending on your preference)

Pinch of cayenne pepper

½ avocado, pitted and peeled

In a small bowl, cover the sun-dried tomatoes with hot water. Allow them to rehydrate, then drain when ready to add them. They should be soft.

In a high-speed blender , combine all the ingredients, including the rehydrated sun-dried tomatoes, but omitting the avocado. Blend until smooth.

Add the avocado and blend again. This soup can be served at room temperature, or let the blender run for several minutes and serve warm.

Adjust the seasoning and flavors to taste and pour into bowls.

Eat right away or store in the fridge for 1 to 2 days.

note:

The avocado is added last so that the soup doesn't turn into a mousse.

## serving suggestions:

- Top the bowls with your choice of diced veggies (tomato, avocado, corn kernels, more cilantro, etc.).

- Add nut & seed crackers as a healthy alternative to tortilla chips!

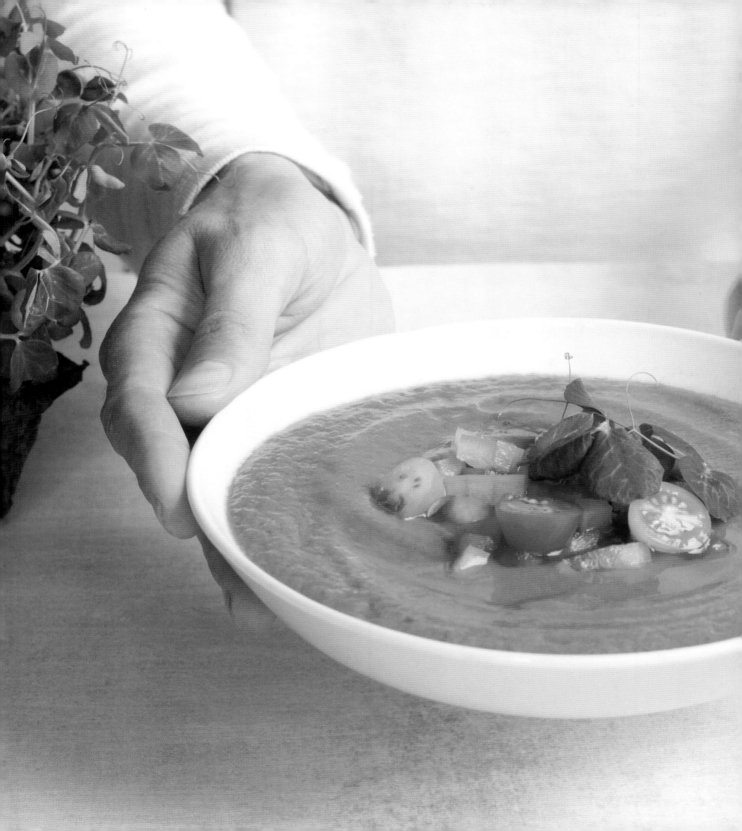

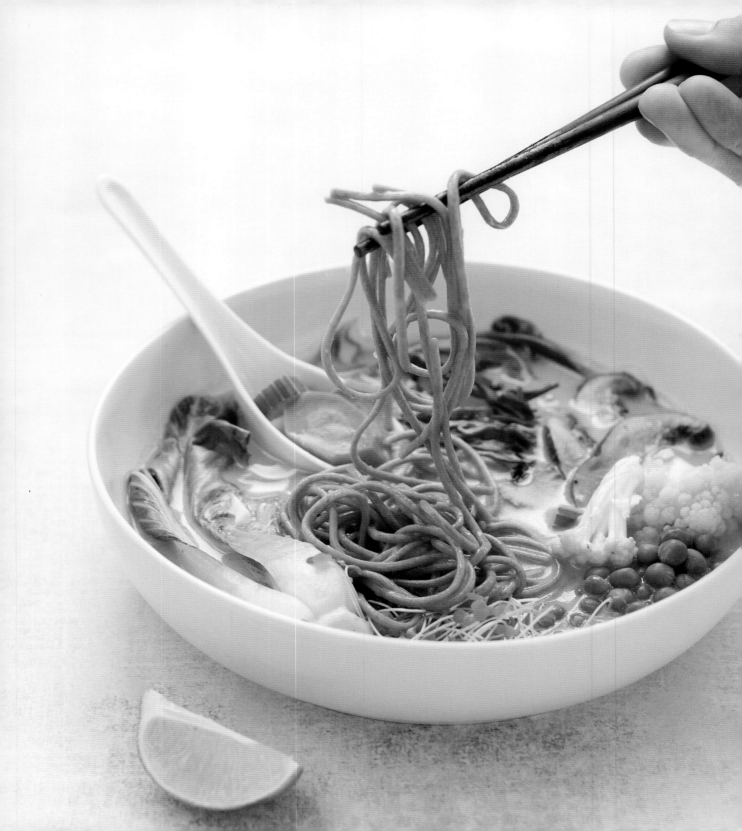

# thai curry ramen

Muscle building | anti-inflammatory | immunity booster • Yields: 2 or 3 servings

Curries are superquick to make and you have total freedom to throw whatever you want into them. This ramen is a perfect dish to make when you have leftover veggies hiding out in the back of your fridge: Just chop them up and toss them in a pan with some coconut milk, herbs and spices. You can enjoy this recipe as is or serve it ramen style. On big training days, we often opt for soba noodles. These noodles are made from buckwheat, which, despite its name, is not wheat at all; it is a gluten-free seed that is a powerhouse of nutrition. Buckwheat is a source of easily digestible high-quality protein with alkaline properties and contains all eight essential amino acids that the body requires to function properly.

¼ cup (40 g) thinly sliced onion

2 tbsp (30 ml) water, plus more if needed

2 cloves garlic, minced

1 (2″ [5-cm]) piece fresh ginger (or more), minced

1 generous tsp ground turmeric

1 tsp yellow curry powder

1 tsp sea salt

1 (13.5-oz [400-ml]) can coconut milk

1 stalk lemongrass, smashed

4 kaffir lime leaves (optional)

4 cups (500 g) chopped fresh mixed veggies (cauliflower, broccoli, carrot, celery, cabbage, etc.)

1 cup (70 g) organic mushrooms, cut into large pieces

⅓ cup (50 g) fresh peas

2 cups (90 g) chopped fresh greens (kale, bok choy, spinach)

**to serve**

2 to 3 cups (240 to 360 g) noodles of choice; such as raw spiralized zucchini squash, cooked 100% buckwheat noodles or lentil noodles

Fresh cilantro or basil, chopped (optional)

2 tbsp (18 g) raw cashews, crushed (optional)

Handful of sprouts (optional)

1 lime, cut into wedges

In a deep medium skillet, sauté the onion in the water for 3 minutes over medium heat. Add the garlic, ginger, turmeric, curry powder and salt and cook for another minute (adding more water if too dry).

Mix in the coconut milk, lemongrass and kaffir lime leaves, if desired. Stir it up and bring to a gentle boil.

Toss in the chopped mixed veggies. Cook for 5 minutes, then add the mushrooms and peas. Lower the heat and simmer, stirring occasionally, for 8 to 10 minutes, or until the veggies are cooked to your preference. When finished cooking, discard the lemongrass and kaffir leaves. Turn the burner off and mix in chopped fresh greens such as kale, bok choy or spinach. Cover the skillet with a lid and allow the curry to sit on a warm stove for a few minutes.

About 10 minutes before serving, prepare your noodles of choice.

To serve, divide the noodles between 2 or 3 serving bowls. Top with the veggie curry and garnish with chopped herbs, raw cashews and sprouts, if desired. Serve with a wedge of lime.

Grab your chopsticks and dig in.

**notes:**

- Kaffir lime leaves are much cheaper bought frozen in Asian supermarkets. They keep well in the freezer until needed.

- If you do not have lemongrass or kaffir lime leaves, you can leave them out. The curry will still taste good.

**pro tip:**

To get maximum nutrition from soba noodles, look for brands made from 100% buckwheat.

# raw pad thai

Raw | alkalizing | thyroid support  •  Soaking time: 2 hours | Yields: 2 servings

If you like the taste of Thai food but don't enjoy the way you feel after eating it, then you will appreciate this dish. It's a nutrient-dense spin on a traditional pad thai that is typically made with rice noodles, egg, some variation of protein and a heavy peanut sauce. In this raw vegan version, we are using zucchini and kelp noodles, carrots, kale and herbs as the base, tossed in a creamy cashew and bell pepper sauce—a great dish to make ahead and pack for a workday lunch.

## noodles

1 (12-oz [340-g]) package kelp noodles (see note)

1 zucchini

⅓ cup (47 g) raw cashews, crushed

1 large carrot, grated

1 cup (90 g) shredded purple cabbage

4 leaves dinosaur kale, thinly chopped

⅓ cup (13 g) fresh cilantro, chopped

2 tbsp (5 g) chopped fresh basil

## sauce

3 tbsp (45 ml) fresh lemon juice

1 cup (140 g) raw cashews, soaked in water for 2 hours and drained

1 red bell pepper, seeded and chopped

2 tbsp (32 g) raw almond butter

1 tbsp (15 ml) purified water

¼ tsp sea salt

## to serve

1 raw, organic nori sheet, thinly sliced or cut with kitchen scissors

1 lime, cut into wedges

Prepare the noodles: Rinse and drain the kelp noodles, then cut them a few times with kitchen scissors to make them smaller.

To make your zucchini noodles, use a spiralizer on the thick noodle setting. If you don't have spiralizer, you can cut the zucchini into long, thin strips or use a potato peeler to get a noodlelike effect.

In a large bowl, combine the kelp and zucchini noodles. Mix in the cashews, carrot, cabbage, kale, cilantro and basil. Set aside.

Prepare the sauce: In a blender, blend together all the sauce ingredients until smooth.

Pour ½ cup (120 ml) of the sauce over the noodles and gently mix in. Add more sauce if needed, until the noodles are thoroughly coated with sauce.

Serve garnished with the nori and lime wedges.

### note:

Kelp noodles are a seaweed-based noodle that is high in iodine, very low in calories, low in carbs and high in fiber. Kelp noodles come in a package and you can buy them at many health food stores or online.

### pro tip:

If you cannot find kelp noodles, you can make this dish without them. Simply add extra zucchini noodles, plus another shredded carrot.

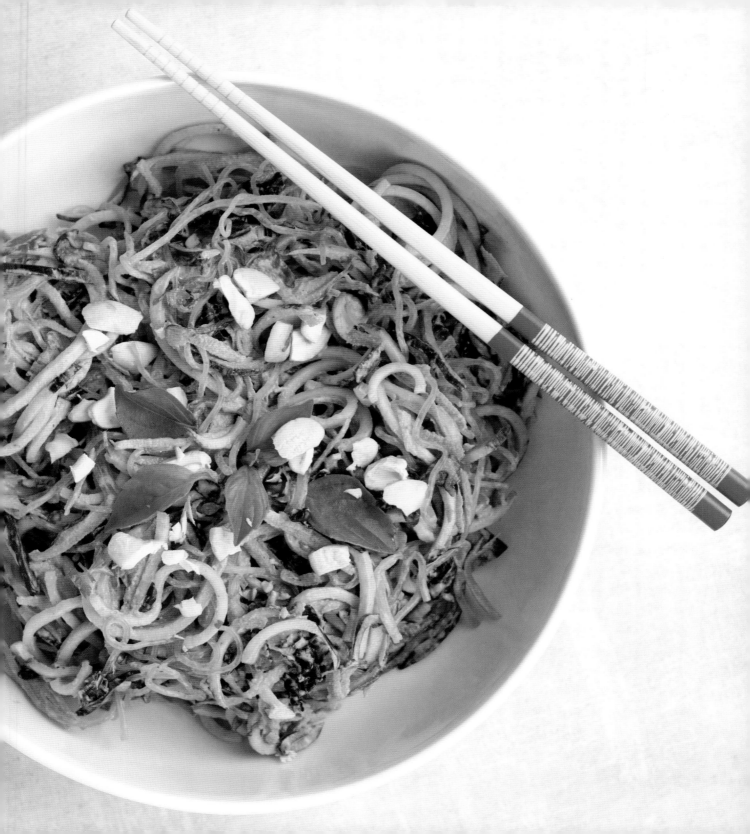

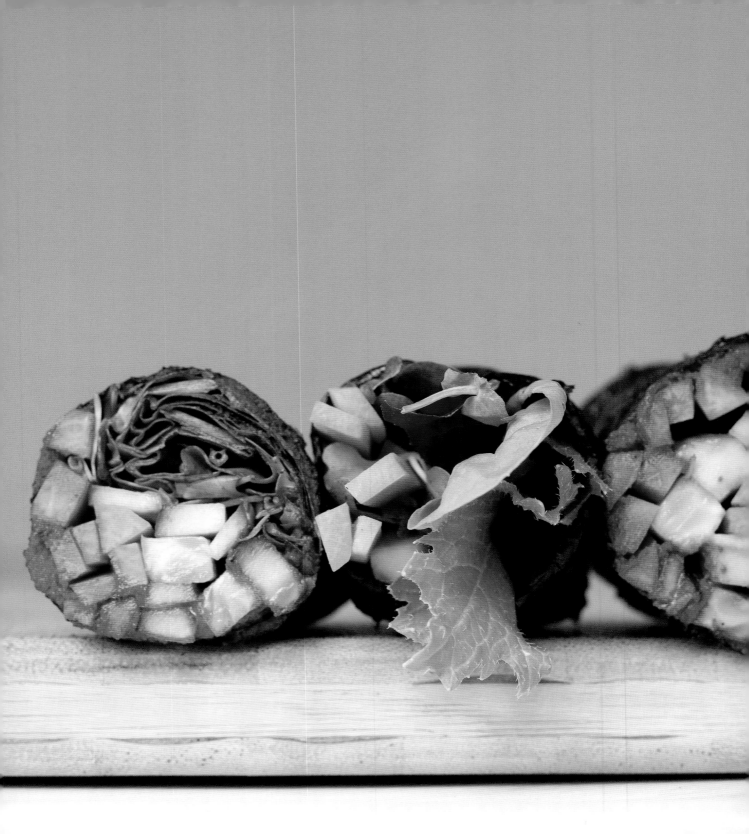

# veggie nori rolls

Mineral rich | detoxifying | thyroid support • Yields: 1 or 2 servings

These veggie rolls make a regular appearance on our dinner table. They are easy to make, don't require much prep and are very satisfying. Think of them as a portable salad. They are perfect for getting extra fresh, raw vegetables and mineral-rich seaweed into your diet. If you have never made sushi rolls at home before, have no fear. It might look fancy; however, it's an easy process, and even though they might not always turn out perfect, that's okay—they still taste amazing!

4 raw, organic nori sheets

½ cup (120 g) Roasted Beet Dip (page 208) or (123 g) hummus

1 large carrot, cut in half and thinly sliced

½ cucumber, cut in half and thinly sliced

½ zucchini, cut in half and thinly sliced

2 cups (110 g) mixed salad greens (or more or less as desired)

Take a nori sheet and spread some beet dip or hummus evenly over it, leaving a narrow uncoated margin around all the edges

Arrange a quarter of the veggies in a level layer along one-half of the dip-coated area, in this order: carrot, cucumber, zucchini and greens.

Starting at the far edge of the veggie side, rolling in parallel with the veggie strips, roll up the nori sheet as tightly as you can, then cut crosswise into 2 to 4 pieces, using a sharp knife. Repeat the process until all the sheets are filled and rolled.

That's how easy it is. Enjoy!

**note:**

Be creative with the filling. You can't really go wrong—use a variety of fresh vegetables you already have on hand and slice them thinly.

**pro tip:**

Veggie rolls make a great portable meal. Prep the night before and pack them for lunch.

# walnut meat lettuce tacos

Raw | anti-inflammatory | brain food • Soaking time: 4 to 8 hours | Yields: 3 or 4 servings

Meet the quickest and healthiest way to satisfy your Mexican food cravings! We believe that every recipe we create should be nutrient-dense and at the same time tasty and enjoyable. These tacos deliver on all those requirements. It's pretty amazing how a few seasonings can transform nuts and mushrooms to taste like meat. For taco shells, we are keeping it clean and simple, using butter lettuce. Add some seasonal fresh veggies, then tie it all together with our Clean Sour Cream (page 200) and you've got yourself an excellent meal that is packed full of nutrients and flavor.

## walnut meat

1 cup (67 g) shiitake mushrooms

2 cups (200 g) raw walnuts, soaked in water for 4 to 8 hours

1 clove garlic

1 tsp ground cumin

1 tsp smoked paprika

½ tsp Himalayan pink salt

## to assemble

1 to 2 heads butter lettuce

1 cup (150 g) cherry tomatoes, sliced

1 cup (116 g) radishes, sliced

1 avocado, peeled, pitted and sliced lengthwise

Handful of fresh cilantro, chopped

¼ cup (56 g) sun-dried black olives, pitted and sliced

Clean Sour Cream (page 200; optional)

Prepare the walnut meat: Wash and dry the mushrooms. In a food processor, combine all the walnut meat ingredients and pulse until a chunky consistency forms.

To assemble the tacos, place 2 to 3 tablespoons (11 to 18 g) of the walnut meat into the center of a lettuce leaf, taco style. Top with tomato, radish, avocado, cilantro, olives and sour cream, if desired. Repeat to assemble the remaining tacos. Once assembled, serve immediately.

Store any leftover walnut meat in a sealed glass container and use within 3 to 4 days.

notes:

- Feel free to replace the butter lettuce with romaine or iceberg lettuce or organic corn tortillas.

- This recipe is very flexible. Feel free to add or remove any toppings or ingredients to suit your needs and taste buds.

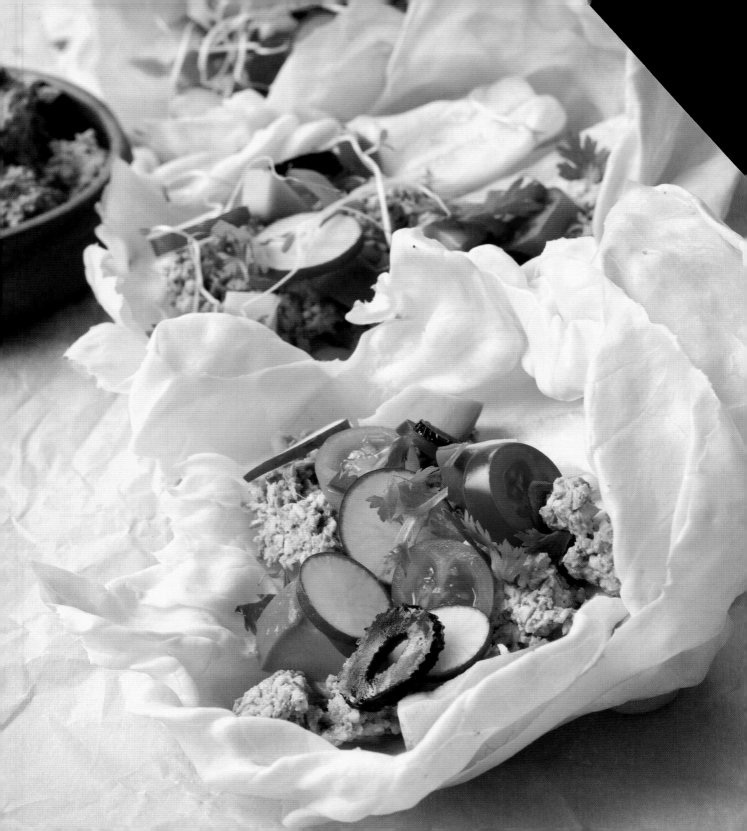

# bowl

...rk this page and refer to it regularly, as this is one of the ultimate go-to ...workout or an active day outdoors. The beauty about Nourish Bowls ...e freedom to embrace your creative side and allow you the flexibility ...l produce as well as utilize any veggies that you have on hand. The ...pt is essentially a colorful, filling dish overflowing a large bowl—composed of whole grains, vegetables (raw, sautéed or roasted), protein (legumes, tempeh), greens, sprouts and seeds—and finished off with a homemade dressing. Depending on which herbs and spices you choose, the dressing will transform each bowl into a unique creation.

## nourish bowl ingredient suggestions

*Whole Grains (1 to 2 parts, uncooked)*

- Quinoa
- Sprouted buckwheat
- Wild rice
- Brown rice
- Amaranth
- Millet
- Soba noodles
- Roasted sweet potato or squash

*Vegetables (1 to 2 parts)*

- Romaine, green or red leaf lettuce
- Kale, Swiss chard, arugula or spinach
- Cabbage (any variety), shredded
- Carrot, thinly sliced or shredded
- Avocado
- Zucchini, chopped or spiralized
- Bell peppers, sliced
- Cucumber
- Radishes
- Tomatoes
- Green beans
- Mushrooms
- Broccoli, cauliflower

*Protein (1 part)*

- Organic tempeh, sliced
- Lentils—green, yellow or red
- Beans—garbanzo (chickpeas), cannellini (white kidney), kidney or black beans
- Organic green peas
- Organic edamame (whole soybeans)
- Nuts or seeds, raw

*Superfood Boost (1 to 2 tbsp [15 to 30 g], except turmeric)*

- Fresh herbs, chopped (cilantro, parsley, mint, basil, chives)
- Sprouts (alfalfa, lentil, broccoli, clover, etc.)
- Goji berries
- Sauerkraut or kimchi
- Seaweed (kelp, dulse or nori)
- Ground turmeric (½ tsp)
- Hemp hearts

## dressing

*Keep it simple*

- Cider vinegar, Balsamic Vinaigrette (page 198), fresh lime or lemon juice, extra virgin olive oil, hemp or flaxseed oil

*Make it fancy*

- Clean Sour Cream (page 200), Lemon-Tahini Sauce (page 199) or Cilantro Chutney (page 201)

Select and cook your grains: Cooking times vary greatly—so if you're cooking on a busy weeknight, pick a quick-cooking grain and start it simmering on the stove first. Another easy approach is to select 1 or 2 grains for the week and make a big batch on Sunday. Cooked grains keep for 5 to 6 days in the fridge.

Prepare all your vegetables of choice: Chop, dice, shred or grate any raw veggies you like and steam or roast such veggies as cauliflower, broccoli and mushrooms.

Prep your protein: Tempeh can be baked in a marinade of equal parts extra virgin olive oil and balsamic vinegar for added flavor. Dried beans and lentils will need to be soaked a day ahead, then simmered for 30 minutes to 2 hours, so plan accordingly—beans and lentils, just like grains, can be made in a big batch on Sunday for the workweek. You can heat them or leave them cold If you're short on time, use canned beans (make sure to drain and rinse thoroughly) or pick up precooked lentils available in many grocery stores.

Superfood your bowl: This step is optional; however, it does add an extra nutritional boost to your meal. Put a handful of fresh herbs or fermented veggies on top of your Nourish Bowl. Sprinkle with some goji berries or hemp hearts. Top with fresh sprouts.

Dress it up: You can either dress your bowl with a simple drizzle of extra virgin olive oil, balsamic vinegar or lemon juice and salt and pepper, or get fancy by choosing one of the sauces/dressings/dips from this book.

Serve and enjoy!

*See photo on page 132.

> **note:**
>
> Nourish bowls are a great way to use up leftovers and quickly feed the whole family. Simply put everything out and let everyone build their own bowl.

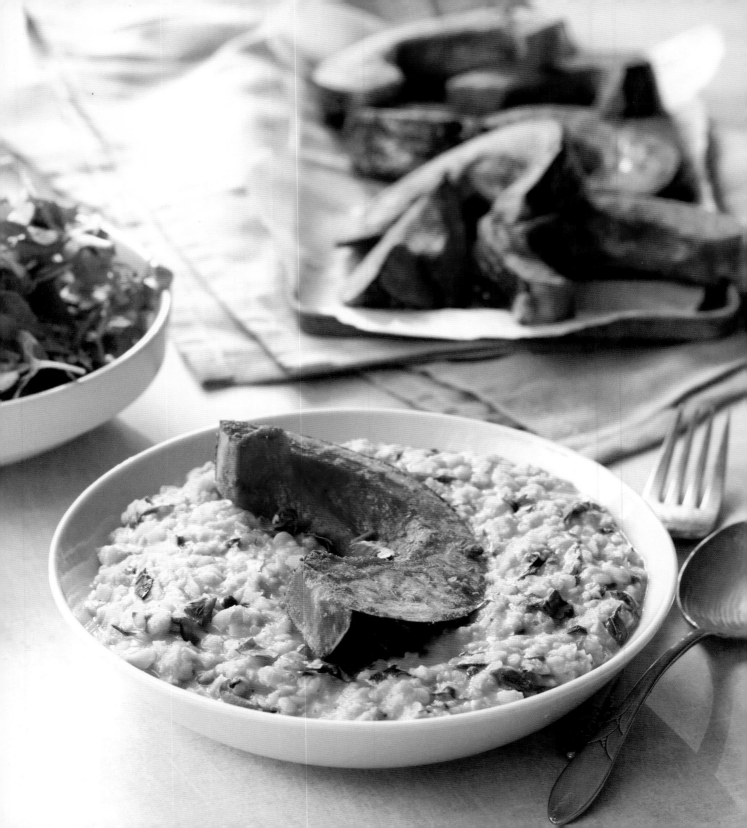

# ayurvedic bowl

*Energizing | protein & iron rich | healing*  •  Yields: 2 servings

Ayurveda is a centuries-old Hindu system of nutrition and medicine that was developed alongside yoga as the best means to prevent illness and imbalance. Far more a lifestyle than a diet, a famous Ayurvedic saying is "When diet is wrong, medicine is of no use; when diet is correct, medicine is of no need." A simple combination of lentils, veggies and calming herbs and spices, this Ayurvedic bowl is easy to digest, and it brings balance and nourishment to the body. We love the roasted kabocha squash here, as it's a lovely addition to this meal and provides beneficial low-glycemic carbohydrates to fuel your long runs, hard workouts or any other intense efforts.

### roasted squash

1 tbsp (15 g) coconut oil

¼ tsp ground cumin

1 tsp mild yellow curry powder

Sea salt and freshly ground black pepper

½ medium kabocha squash, seeded and cut into wedges

### dal

¾ cup (169 g) red lentils, soaked in water for 4 to 8 hours

2 tbsp (30 ml) water, plus more if needed

¼ medium red onion, finely diced

¼ tsp sea salt

2 tsp (4 g) mild yellow curry powder

¼ tsp ground cumin

1 (1" [2.5-cm]) piece fresh ginger, peeled and grated

1 (13.5-oz [400-ml]) can full-fat coconut milk

4 leaves Swiss chard, chopped

Prepare the squash: Preheat the oven to 400°F (200°C) and line a baking sheet with parchment paper.

In a large bowl, combine the coconut oil, cumin, curry powder, salt and pepper to taste. Toss the squash pieces in the mixture to coat, then spread out the squash in a single layer on the prepared baking sheet. Roast until browned and tender, about 35 minutes.

Prepare the dal: Drain and rinse the soaked lentils and set aside.

In a small saucepan, heat the 2 tablespoons (30 ml) of water. Add the onion and salt and cook, stirring, until softened, 3 to 5 minutes. Add the curry powder, cumin and ginger and cook, stirring, for a couple of minutes more, until very fragrant. Add the lentils and coconut milk. Cook, frequently stirring, for 10 to 12 minutes, until the lentils are tender and the dal is thick, adding a little bit of water if needed to obtain your desired consistency. Stir in the chard, turn off the heat and let it sit for 3 minutes.

Divide the dal between 2 bowls and top with a couple of pieces of roasted squash to serve.

## serving suggestions:

Garnish with chopped fresh cilantro and serve with a side of Green Mix Salad (page 59).

## pro tip:

Although this recipe only calls for half of one squash, go ahead and roast the whole thing. You can easily use it through the week by incorporating it into your salad or grain bowls, or enjoy a couple of pieces as a preworkout snack.

# quinoa bowl

...me one of your new favorite go-to meals. Ready in just about 15 minutes
...cold, it's perfect for a quick weeknight dinner, potluck or picnic. You can
...a big batch and bring it into work throughout the week, too.

½ cup (28 g) sun-dried tomatoes, chopped

**quinoa**

1 cup (173 g) uncooked quinoa

2 cups (475 ml) water

Pinch of salt

**pesto**

1 very ripe avocado

1 cup (60 g) fresh parsley or (40 g) basil leaves

¼ cup (25 g) walnuts

1 clove garlic

1 (½" [1.3-cm]) piece fresh ginger, peeled and chopped

Juice of ½ lemon

¼ tsp Celtic sea salt

**bowl**

Handful of baby spinach

1 to 2 tbsp (11 to 22 g) hemp hearts, for sprinkling

In a small bowl cover the sun-dried tomatoes with hot water. Allow them to rehydrate while you get the rest of the recipe ready.

Prepare the quinoa: Rinse, drain and then place the quinoa in a medium saucepan along with the water and salt. Bring the quinoa to a boil, cover with a tight-fitting lid, lower the heat and allow to simmer for 15 minutes.

While the quinoa cooks, prepare the pesto: Halve the avocado, remove the pit and scoop out the pulp. In a food processor or blender, combine the avocado, parsley, walnuts and garlic and blend until smooth.

Add the ginger, lemon juice and salt and pulse for few more seconds, or until creamy.

Assemble the bowl: Drain the sun-dried tomatoes and place them in a large bowl. Add the cooked quinoa and pesto and stir well. After the quinoa has slightly cooled, add the spinach (it will wilt if the quinoa is too hot).

Sprinkle the hemp hearts on top and serve.

## pro tips:

- Leftover pesto is excellent for quick weekday meals. You can use it instead of dressings on salads or zucchini noodles or spread it on sprouted-grain toast; it also makes a great dip for flax crackers and fresh veggies. Store leftover pesto in a glass jar with a tight-fitting lid and use within 2 days.

- Cooked quinoa should be fluffy and slightly chewy, but never crunchy. If you end up with leftovers, you can store it in the fridge for up to 3 days. It's a great addition to your salads; it also makes the perfect morning cereal when mixed with fresh berries and your plant-based milk of choice.

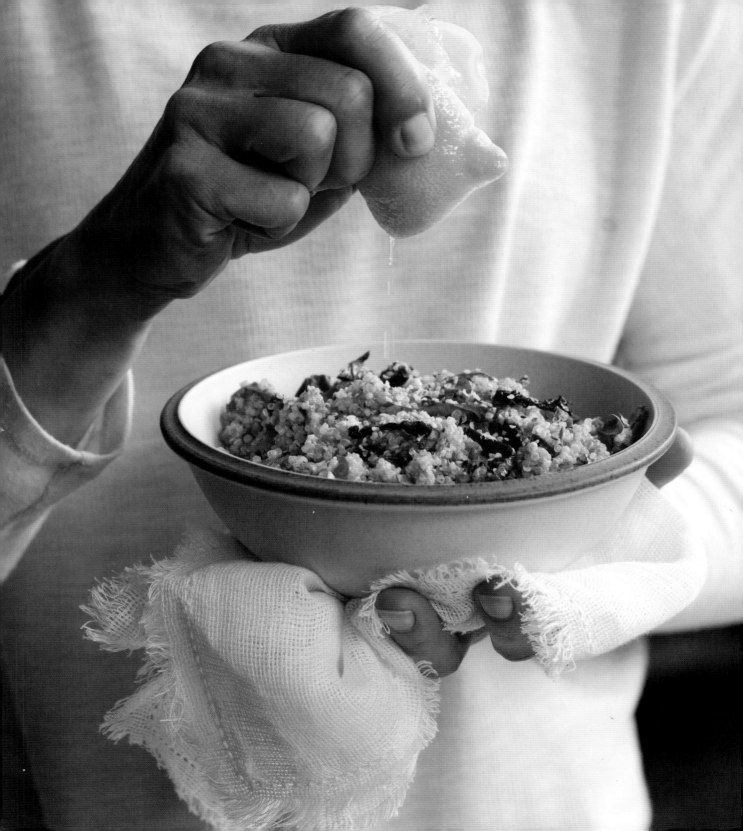

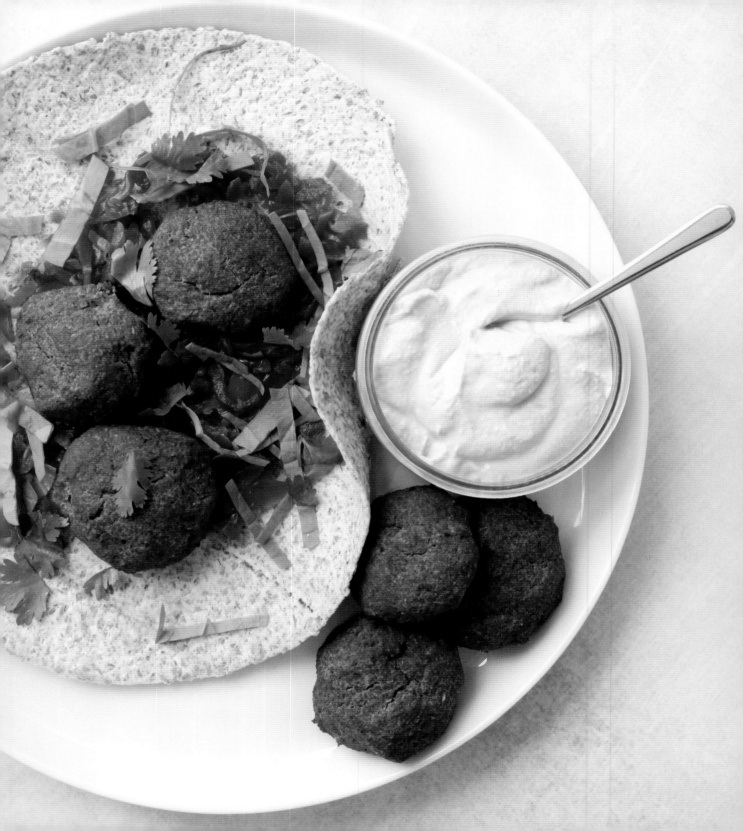

# sprouted falafel

Raw option | protein and iron rich • Soaking time: 20 minutes | Yields: 24 to 28 pieces

A delicious crispy falafel made with sprouted chickpeas instead of cooked. Chickpeas are a great way to add a complete protein to your plant-powered diet. They are full of fiber and trace minerals; they are also low glycemic and a good source of iron. Once your chickpeas are sprouted, this recipe comes together in about 30 minutes and makes a large batch that can be saved for easy weeknight meals or snacks on the run. Their high protein and fiber content makes these falafel filling for lasting energy. Two or three patties can be a hearty meal, especially if eaten with a big green salad.

2½ cups (412 g) sprouted chickpeas (see note)

1 cup (55 g) sun-dried tomatoes, soaked in water for 20 minutes

½ cup (120 g) tahini

5 ribs celery, chopped

Juice of 1 lemon

3 cloves garlic, peeled

1 tsp ground cumin

1 tsp ground coriander

1 tsp Celtic sea salt

⅓ cup (80 ml) coconut aminos or nama shoyu

¼ cup (15 g) fresh parsley, chopped

¼ cup (10 g) fresh cilantro, chopped

¼ cup (28 g) flax meal

Olive oil, for brushing (if baking)

In a food processor, combine the sprouted chickpeas, sun-dried tomatoes, tahini, celery, lemon juice, garlic, cumin, coriander, salt and coconut aminos and process until well mixed. You want a crumbly dough, not a smooth paste, adding a little water if needed.

Transfer the mixture to a bowl, add the parsley, cilantro and flax meal and mix well.

Form a golf ball–sized portion of the falafel mixture into a small patty, using your hands. Repeat until all the patties are formed.

## cooked

Preheat the oven to 375°F (190°C). Line a baking sheet with parchment paper.

Brush the top of each falafel with olive oil and bake, turning every 5 minutes, until the falafel are evenly browned, about 20 minutes.

## raw

Place the falafel on the mesh screen of a dehydrator tray.

Dehydrate for 6 hours at 115°F (46°C). You can turn them partway through that period. Falafel should be dry and slightly crisp on the outside and still moist on the inside.

The falafel will keep in an airtight container for 5 to 7 days in the refrigerator or up to 4 weeks in the freezer.

## serving suggestions:

- You can eat these on their own as an appetizer or snack.
- Put them on top of the Green Mix Salad (page 59) or Nourish Bowl (page 146).
- Add to a sprouted-grain pita or collard wrap with some hummus, Mango Salsa (page 204), Lemon-Tahini Sauce (page 199) and fresh or roasted vegetables.

### note:

Although using canned beans might seem more convenient, they are known to cause digestive upset, such as bloating and gas. Instead, take the extra step and sprout your chickpeas. Sprouting is very easy and significantly reduces the amount of phytic acid in the chickpeas, which means more nourishment for you. Details on sprouting can be found on page 27.

# greek-style spaghetti squash

Easy to digest | iron rich | pre- & postworkout fuel  •  Soaking time: 8 hours
| Yields: 2 servings

This recipe is a healthy spin on a meal we enjoyed while visiting the island of Crete several years ago. Traditionally made with pasta, this gluten-free variation uses spaghetti squash instead of noodles. Mediterranean-style herbs, caramelized onion and good-quality olives make this an amazingly flavorful meal. Spaghetti squash is a versatile low-calorie vegetable that supplies complex carbohydrates needed to fuel long runs, hard workouts and other intense training sessions. A dish like this one is also an excellent choice as part of a postworkout recovery meal. The body's muscles and other tissues need to be replenished with carbohydrates paired with some protein; the combination of fiber-rich vegetables and easy-to-digest lentils is a perfect option due to its overall nutritional package.

1 (3-lb [1.4-kg]) spaghetti squash

½ cup (113 g) dried green lentils, soaked in water for 8 hours, or 1 cup (198 g) cooked

½ cup (80 g) thinly sliced red onion

2 cloves garlic, minced

2 tbsp (30 ml) cider vinegar

1 bell pepper, any color, seeded and diced

1 tbsp (6 g) dried Mediterranean herb mix or any combination of rosemary, oregano, marjoram, za'atar, thyme and sage

1 tsp sea salt

1 cup (150 g) cherry tomatoes, halved

½ cup (30 g) fresh parsley, chopped

¼ cup (25 g) raw black olives, pitted and sliced (see pro tip)

1 tsp capers (optional)

Freshly ground black pepper

## pro tip:

Avoid using low-quality canned olives or gourmet-style olives. Instead, look for sun-ripened black olives without any dyes.

Preheat the oven to 350°F (180°C). Cut the spaghetti squash in half lengthwise. Scrape out and discard the seeds and membranes. Place the halves, cut side down, in a large baking dish and add ½ cup (120 ml) of water. Bake for 45 to 50 minutes, or until tender.

Meanwhile, if using dried lentils, rinse them well after soaking and place in a saucepan in 1 cup (240 ml) of water. Cook, covered over medium heat for 20 to 30 minutes, adding more water as needed to make sure the lentils are just barely covered. Once tender and no longer crunchy, remove from the heat and set aside.

Remove the squash from the oven. Turn the squash halves cut side up and let cool for 10 minutes. Then, using a fork, scrape out the spaghetti squash strands. If your squash is very moist, you might have to place the strands in a colander and pat them dry with a clean cloth or kitchen towel.

Place the squash strands in a large glass bowl. Gently mix in the lentils.

In a medium skillet, heat 2 tablespoons (30 ml) of water over medium-high heat. Add the red onion and garlic and sauté for 4 minutes. Add the cider vinegar and cook for 5 more minutes, or until the onion is nicely browned.

Lower the heat to medium-low and mix in the bell pepper, Mediterranean herbs and salt. Cook for another 4 minutes before gently stirring into the squash mixture.

Toss in the cherry tomatoes, parsley, olives and capers (if using). Sprinkle with black pepper and serve.

### note:
Use any leftovers for an easy "pack and go" lunch during your workday.

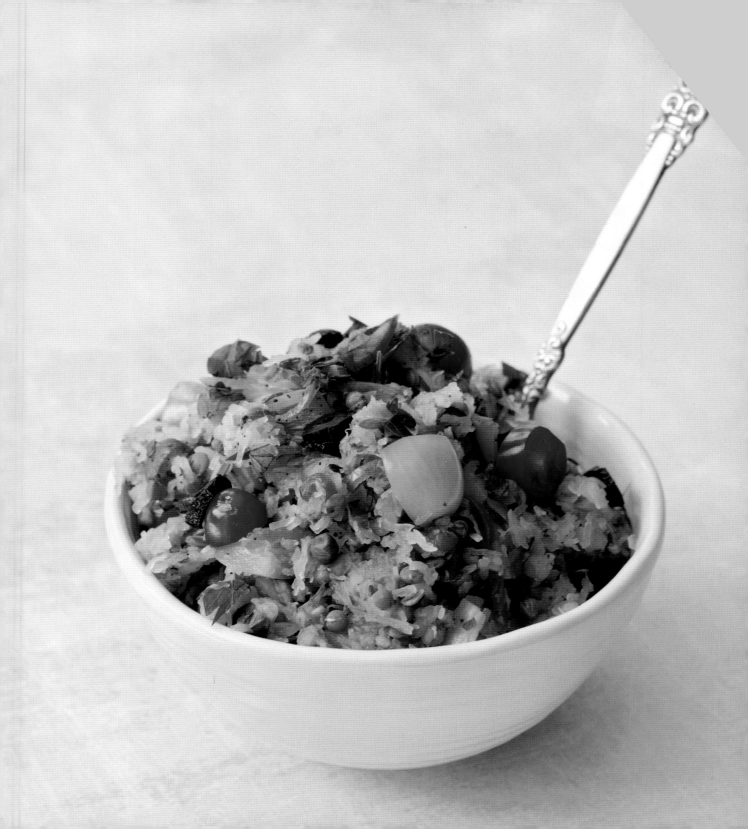

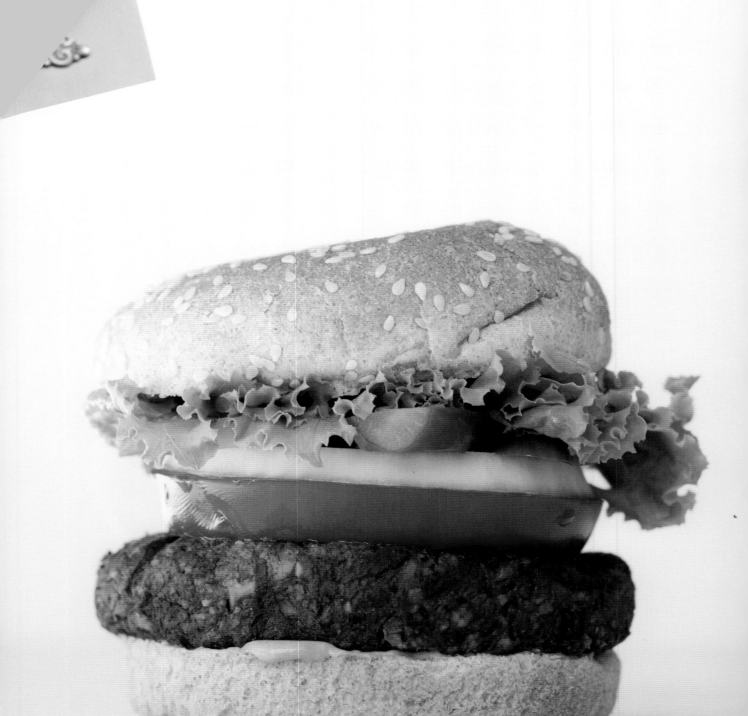

# "the game changer" burger

Muscle building | high fiber | increases bone density  • Soaking time: 8 hours or overnight | Yields: 4 patties

There are a gazillion meat substitute products out there, but since our goal is to nourish our body with the best food possible, we stay away from all ultraprocessed and nutrient-depleted "Frankenfoods." Instead, we eat a whole bunch of vegetables. Also, we sometimes even re-create classic dishes entirely from these beautiful, nourishing plants—such as this veggie burger, made totally from scratch using only high-quality ingredients. It feels so natural to eat this way—so obvious that this is how we are supposed to eat. Give this veggie burger a try; it won't disappoint you. Oh, and did I mention each burger has nearly 13 grams of protein?!

¾ cup (75 g) walnuts, soaked in water for 8 hours or overnight

1 tbsp (14 g) coconut oil, plus more to cook patties

½ sweet onion, chopped

2 cloves garlic, minced

1 cup (70 g) mushrooms, washed and chopped

½ (8-oz [225-g]) package tempeh, crumbled

1 tbsp (7 g) ground flaxseeds

¼ tsp sea salt

¼ tsp freshly ground pepper

½ tsp smoked paprika

1 tbsp (15 ml) coconut aminos or nama shoyu

½ cup (113 g) shredded beet

Drain and rinse the soaked walnuts; set aside.

Heat a medium skillet over medium heat. Once hot, add the oil, onion, garlic and mushrooms and sauté for 3 to 4 minutes, or until the onion is fragrant, soft and translucent. Remove from the heat and transfer the mixture to a food processor or blender. Add the walnuts, tempeh, flaxseeds, salt, pepper, smoked paprika and coconut aminos. Process until well combined but still grainy.

Transfer the mixture to a large bowl and mix in the shredded beet. Set aside for about 15 minutes, so the flax can soak up the liquid and the mixture sets (this step is important for the patties to hold together).

Lightly oil a medium skillet with coconut oil and heat over medium heat.

Meanwhile, shape the burger mixture into 4 patties and arrange as many as you can in the skillet without overcrowding. Cook the patties for about 4 minutes on each side, until lightly browned. Cook any remaining patties in the same manner.

## serving suggestions:

- Serve warm on sprouted-grain buns with chosen toppings.
- For a grain-free meal, crumble a patty on top of Green Mix Salad (page 59) and dress with Balsamic Vinaigrette (page 198).

## pro tip:

The patties are wonderful to cook completely ahead of time and then store in a sealed container in your fridge or freezer. Then, when the urge hits you . . . have at it!

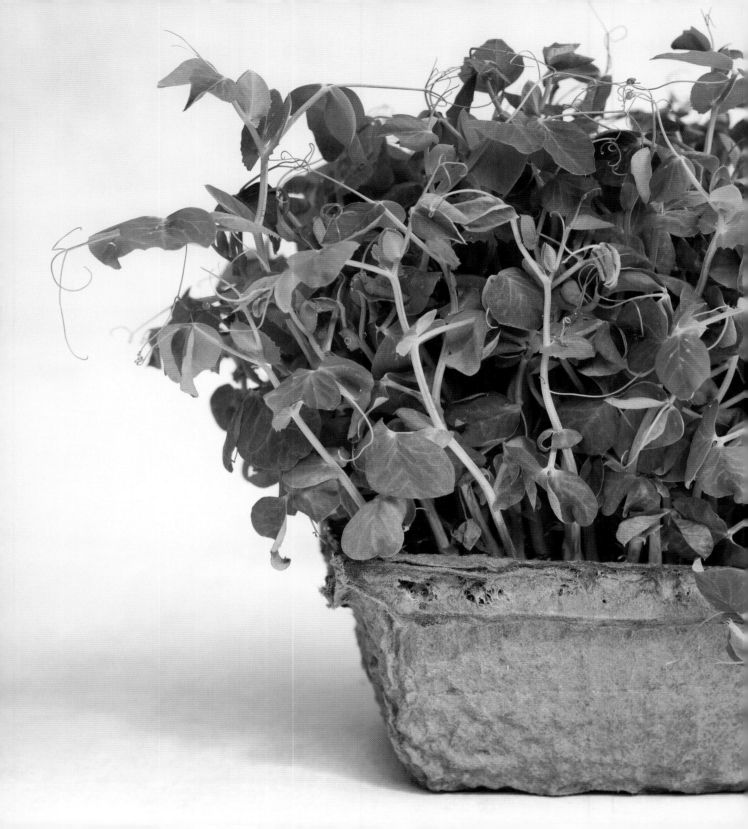

# super salads

To support your athletic performance and recover faster after challenging workouts, eat a big salad each day! The following main dish salads are quick and easy to toss together, overflowing with ultrafresh veggies, and the right amount of nutrients to support your health and fitness goals. From the light yet satisfying Bok Choy Salad with Citrus-Hemp Dressing (page 161) to the protein-rich Roasted Vegetable & Lentil Salad (page 170), you will find a tasty way to include those powerful veggies into your every day.

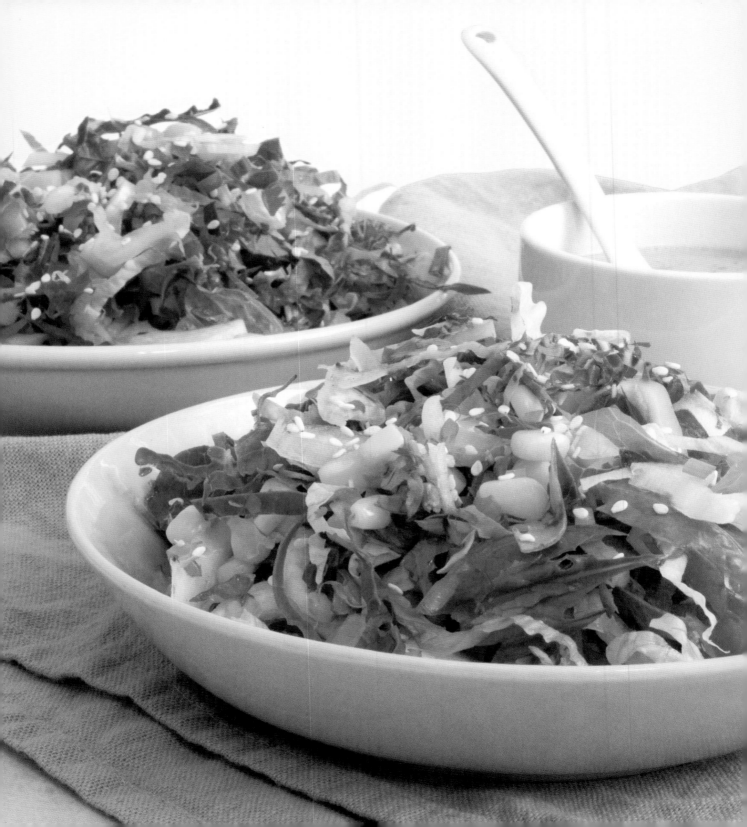

# bok choy salad with citrus-hemp dressing

Raw | bone strengthening | vitamin C rich   •   Yields: 2 servings

Inspired by "Life Regenerator" Dan McDonald, this salad is epic. Bok choy has numerous antioxidants that are powerful cancer fighters, which remain more potent when eaten raw. Do give this salad a try! I am confident it will convince you to add baby bok choy to your rotation of simple green salad options, throughout the summer and beyond.

## salad

1 cup (150 g) fresh, or (130 g) frozen corn, thawed

3 heads baby bok choy

1 small head romaine lettuce

½ cup (20 g) fresh cilantro

1 tbsp (11 g) hemp hearts, for garnish

## dressing

Juice of 2 small oranges

Juice of ½ lemon

1 tbsp (15 ml) cider vinegar

¼ cup (44 g) hemp hearts

2 cloves garlic, peeled

1 (1" [2.5-cm]) piece ginger, peeled

½ tsp Himalayan pink salt

1 tbsp (3 g) dulse flakes

Prepare the salad: Place the raw corn (or thawed frozen corn) in some hot water for a few minutes and then drain.

Personally, I like to run the veggies through a food processor equipped with the slicing blade; however, you can also thinly chop all the greens by hand. Place the chopped bok choy, romaine and cilantro in a large bowl. Add the corn kernels.

Prepare the dressing: In a high-speed blender, combine all the dressing ingredients. Blend until smooth.

Pour the dressing over the veggies and toss well. You can serve right away, but the flavors get even better if you let the salad sit for 20 to 30 minutes, tossing every now and then.

When ready to serve, garnish each serving with 1½ teaspoons (6 g) of hemp hearts.

### note:

Always use organic corn! Buying 100% organic, certified organic, or "USDA Organic"–labeled products are usually the easiest way to avoid genetically modified ingredients.

### pro tips:

- The easiest way to clean baby bok choy is to treat it like a bunch of celery. Trim off and discard the end of the bulb and separate the stalks. Wash the stalks in cool water, carefully brushing away any sand or dirt that remains.
- This salad gets better if it sits for a bit, which makes it a great salad for workday lunches. A bonus: Thanks to the sturdy bok choy and corn, it doesn't get soggy.

# garden salad with sumac vinaigrette

Raw | high in antioxidants | bone health  •  Yields: 2 servings

This colorful salad is an invitation for you to get creative in the kitchen using ingredients from your local farmers' market or garden. The light vinaigrette is the real star of this salad. Sumac, a dried red spice with a tangy, slightly fruity flavor, used traditionally in Middle Eastern cuisine, is rich in antioxidants, and its potential health benefits include decreased cholesterol levels, lower blood sugar, reduced bone loss and relief from muscle pain.

## dressing

Juice of 1 lemon

1 tbsp (15 ml) cider vinegar

2 tbsp (30 ml) extra virgin olive oil

1 tbsp (15 ml) agave nectar

1 tbsp (6 g) minced or grated fresh ginger

½ tsp sumac powder

½ tsp ground cumin

Salt and freshly ground black pepper

## salad

½ medium cucumber, chopped

1 small zucchini, chopped

1 bell pepper, seeded and chopped

2 small carrots, chopped

1 cup (150 g) cherry tomatoes, halved

½ cup (20 g) fresh parsley, finely chopped

2 tbsp (5 g) finely chopped fresh mint

Prepare the dressing: In a large bowl, mix together all the dressing ingredients, including the salt and black pepper to taste.

Prepare the salad: Add the cucumber, zucchini, bell pepper, carrots, tomatoes and herbs to the bowl and mix everything thoroughly until the vinaigrette covers all the vegetables.

Serve!

**note:**

If you can't find it or don't have sumac, you can replace it with fresh lemon zest.

## pro tip:

This salad tastes even better if you let it sit for a while. For this reason, it makes a great option for your workday lunches; make it the night before, refrigerate overnight and enjoy the next day!

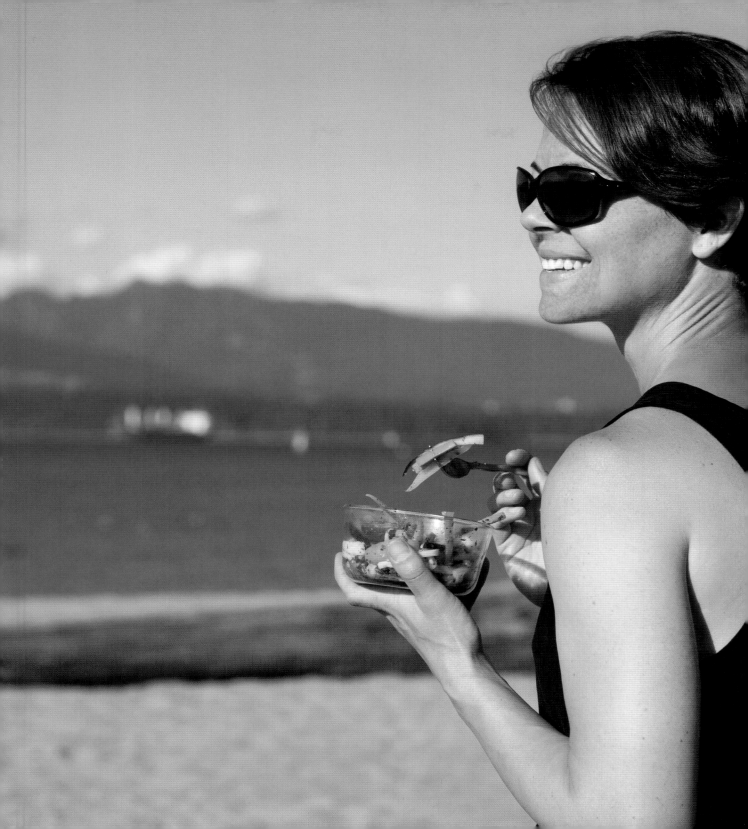

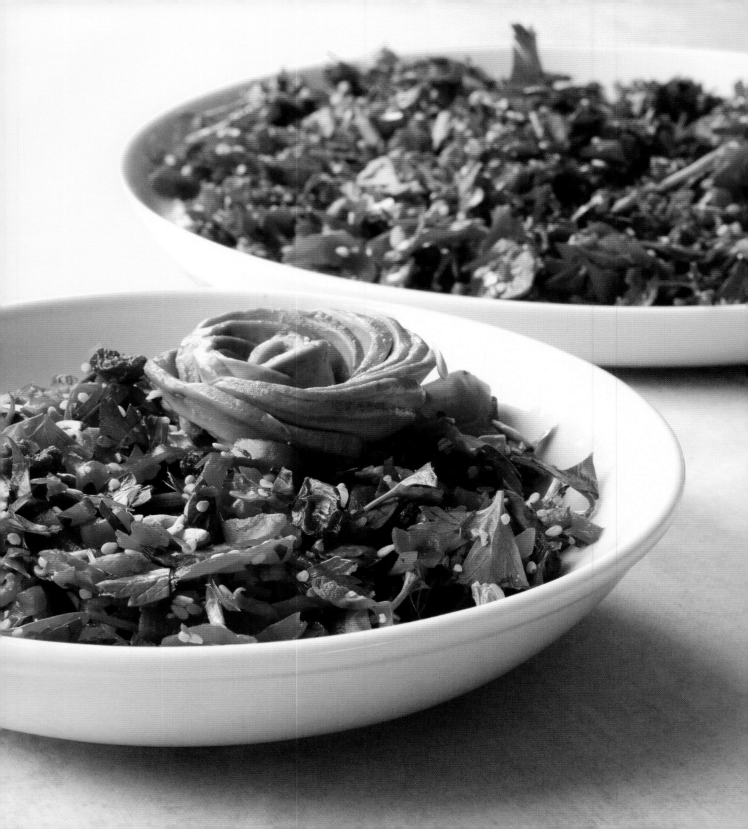

# detox salad

Raw | liver strengthening | detoxifying • Yields: 2 servings

Getting nutrients into your body and getting toxins out is one of the primary ways to ensure great health and maximize your performance. A simple way to start eliminating toxins and enhance your body's ability to absorb nutrients is by adding fermented foods such as sauerkraut into your diet. This detox-friendly salad, apart from being rich in probiotics that help rebalance your gastrointestinal health, is also jam-packed with nutrients to support your body's overall detoxification system. It requires very little work, not much more than placing a few delicious and healing ingredients in one bowl, and it can be made ahead of time to fit into your busy schedule.

2 cups (284 g) purple sauerkraut (see notes)

1 bunch flat-leaf parsley, roughly chopped

¼ cup (40 g) mixed seeds (pumpkin, sunflower, sesame, hemp)

2 tbsp (18 g) raisins, rinsed

1 avocado, peeled, pitted and sliced

In a large bowl, combine the sauerkraut, parsley, seeds and raisins and toss until well combined. To serve, transfer to smaller bowls or plates and top each serving with half of the sliced avocado.

The salad will keep for up to 3 days in the fridge.

**notes:**

- Whenever possible, use homemade sauerkraut (page 67).
- If you're purchasing sauerkraut from a supermarket, make sure that it hasn't been pasteurized (unpasteurized is typically found in the refrigerated section of the store). When heat is applied to food (and this happens with many commercial brands), the beneficial probiotics/bacteria will be damaged, and this then defeats the whole point of eating fermented foods.

# greek salad in a jar

High in antioxidants | muscle meal | rich in B vitamins   •   Yields: 4 servings

Only recently we hopped on the salad-in-a-jar bandwagon. As it turns out, they're the perfect, portable solution for getting in your veggies while on the go, plus you can make four or five at a time—enough to get you through the entire workweek without having to chop and assemble your salad ingredients every day. That's a win-win situation! Although any type of salad certainly works here, this Greek salad—loaded with tomatoes, cucumbers, sun-dried olives and protein-rich quinoa—is perfectly suited for getting packed in a jar. The great thing about this salad is that the lemony vinaigrette keeps its place on the bottom of the jar, while all the other ingredients get layered and packed on top, so everything stays dressing-free until you toss the salad in a bowl. If you don't have all the listed ingredients that's okay. Just use whatever produce you have on hand.

## salad

1 cup (173 g) uncooked quinoa

1 cucumber, diced

2 cups (300 g) cherry tomatoes, halved

2 bell peppers, seeded and chopped

½ cup (50 g) walnuts, chopped

¼ cup (56 g) sun-dried black olives, sliced

4 cups (220 g) chopped mixed greens (romaine is great, too)

## dressing

¼ cup (60 ml) extra virgin olive oil

½ cup (120 ml) fresh lemon juice

1 tbsp (15 ml) Dijon mustard

3 cloves garlic, minced, or 2 tsp (6 g) garlic powder

¼ cup (10 g) basil, finely chopped, or 1 tbsp (2 g) dried

1 tbsp (4 g) chopped fresh oregano, or 1 tsp dried

Himalayan pink salt and freshly ground black pepper (about ¼ tsp each)

Begin the salad: Cook the quinoa according to the package directions. Set aside to cool.

Meanwhile, prepare the dressing: In a small jar or other container with a lid, combine all the dressing ingredients. Screw the lid on the jar and shake to combine.

Assemble the salad: Add 1 to 4 tablespoons (15 to 60 ml) of dressing to the bottom of each jar, depending on personal preference.

Add the cucumber, cooked quinoa, tomatoes, bell peppers, walnuts and olives. Finish by adding the chopped mixed greens to fill the jar.

Screw the lid on the jar and store the salad in the refrigerator for up to 4 days.

When you're ready to eat, unscrew the lid and pour the salad into a bowl. As you do so, the dressing will coat the ingredients. If not, use your fork to gently toss the salad.

Now, of course, you don't have to put the salad in a jar. Place all the prepped components in a large salad bowl, toss and serve.

## pro tips:

• Any canning jar can be used, but wide-mouth pint-sized (500-ml) jars are the easiest for both packing the salad and shaking it out.

• Keep in mind these are versatile, so you can swap out anything you don't like for something else or leave it out entirely. A general rule to follow: Dressing always goes in first, lettuce last.

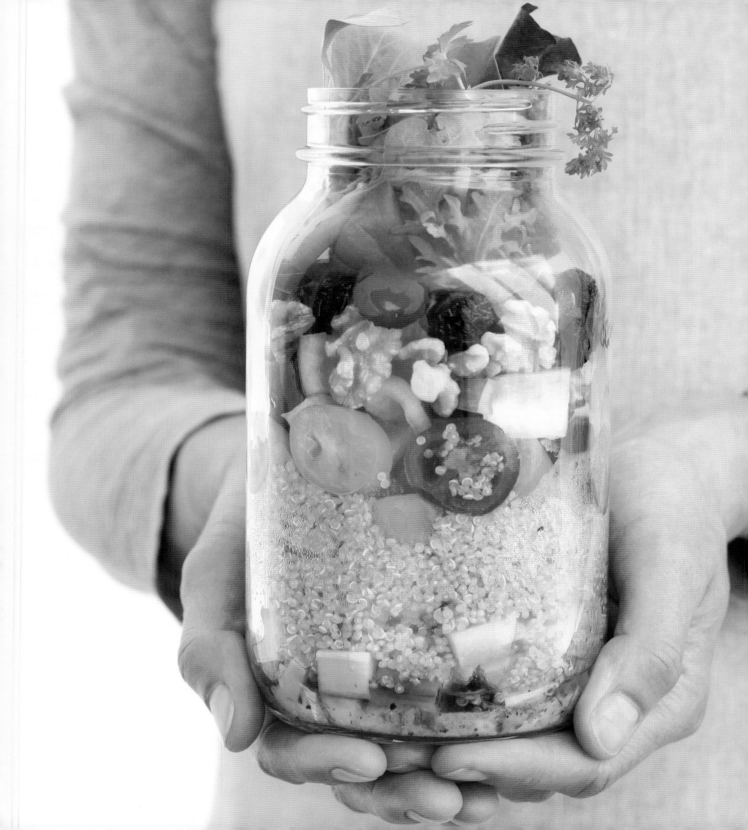

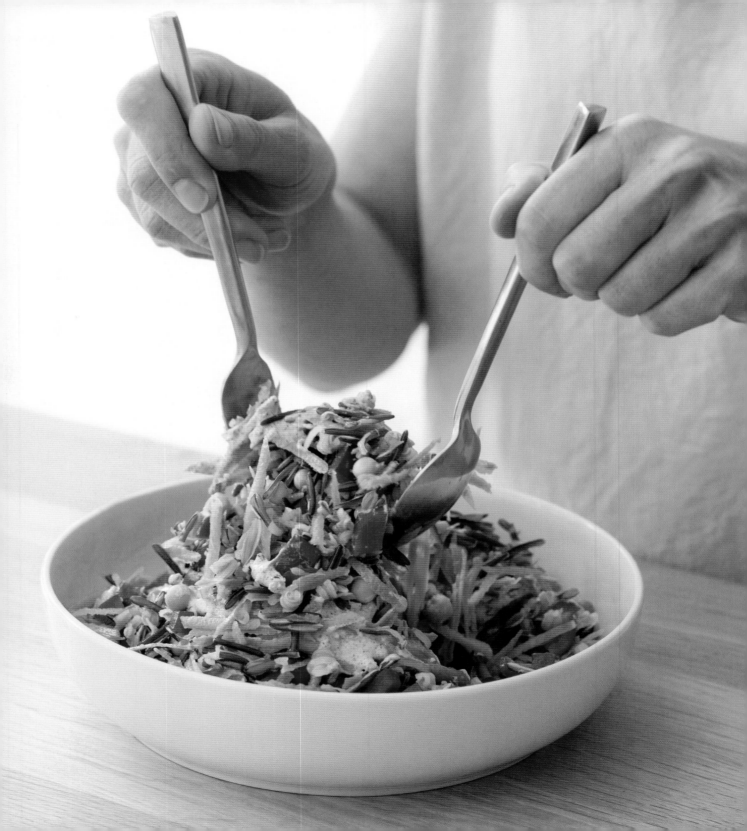

# wild rice salad with creamy miso dressing

Raw option | muscle building | boosts energy   •   Soaking time: overnight (cashews) / 2 to 3 days (rice) | Yields: 2 servings

This salad is well balanced and filling, packing 16 grams of plant-based protein per serving! Wild rice is a grass and is unrefined. It has twice the protein of brown rice; it contains more fiber, potassium and zinc; and offers a wonderful, nutty flavor that works perfectly in salads, soups and Nourish Bowls (page 146). You could either sprout or cook wild rice, keeping in mind that it takes a bit longer to prepare than most grains, so plan accordingly. But it's totally worth it. If your schedule is extra tight, you can always cook this the night before and all you have to do is stir the rest of the ingredients in the last minute.

## salad

½ cup (80 g) uncooked wild rice

½ cup (75 g) fresh or (65 g) frozen peas

1 red bell pepper, seeded and diced

2 carrots, shredded

## dressing

¼ cup (35 g) cashews, soaked in water overnight and drained

¼ cup (36 g) sesame seeds or (60 g) tahini

1 raw, organic nori sheet, torn into pieces

1½ tsp (9 g) organic miso

Juice of 1 lemon

¾ cup (175 ml) purified water, or more

Sea salt and freshly ground black pepper

### note:

If the only wild rice available at your local store is part of a blend, be sure to look for one that is a mix of wild rice and long-grain brown rice, so that the cooking time will be similar.

## cooked

Prepare the salad: Start by rinsing the wild rice well before you cook it, to remove any particles. Bring ¾ cup (175 ml) of water to a boil, add the rice, cover and lower the heat to medium-low.

Cook for 50 to 60 minutes, or until the rice has split open. Every stove cooks differently, so if you still have some water left, just drain it.

While the rice is cooking, if using frozen peas, soak them in 1 cup (240 ml) of warm water for 10 minutes. Set aside.

Prepare the dressing: In a high-speed blender, combine all the dressing ingredients, adding salt and black pepper to taste, and blend until smooth.

Assemble the salad: Place the cooked wild rice in a large bowl. Mix in the bell pepper, carrots and drained green peas. Dress generously with the miso dressing and toss.

## raw

Wild rice takes 2 to 3 days to "bloom" or open, creating an easily digestible raw sprouted base for this salad.

Prepare the salad: Start by rinsing the rice well and placing in a glass bowl or jar with fresh water. Allow to soak at room temperature overnight. The next day, drain and rinse the rice and cover with fresh water. Place in the fridge. Drain, rinse and replenish the water at least once per day until the rice has "bloomed" and becomes tender; this will take 2 to 3 days. Drain, rinse and redrain the rice, then continue with the above recipe directions, skipping the cooking process.

## pro tip:

The salad holds up well if you need to make it in advance. If you do make it ahead of time, add the dressing just before serving.

# roasted vegetable & lentil salad

Protein & iron rich | muscle building  •  Soaking time: 2 hours (optional) | Yields: 2 servings

If you get tired of green salads, try rotating this recipe into the mix. It is a perfect meal to enjoy 1 to 3 hours after your workout or for dinner the night before an endurance race or training session. Lentils are naturally rich in fiber and also a dense source of protein, vitamins and minerals. Together with roasted carrots, beets, mushrooms and a few Indian spices, they create an amazing flavorful meal that will help you replenish or charge you up for a great performance.

4 carrots, scrubbed and trimmed

1 beet, scrubbed and trimmed

2 cups (134 g) shiitake mushrooms, rinsed and dried

2 tbsp (30 ml) extra virgin olive oil

2 cloves garlic, minced

1 tsp garam masala

Sea salt and freshly ground black pepper to taste

½ cup (113 g) dried green lentils, soaked in water for 2 hours, or 1 cup (198 g) cooked

2 cups (40 g) arugula

Preheat the oven to 400°F (200°C) and line a baking sheet with parchment paper.

Halve the carrots lengthwise (if small) or cut into ½-inch (1.3-cm) slices (if large) and quarter the beet.

In a large bowl, combine the carrots, beet and mushrooms. Drizzle with the olive oil, add the garlic, sprinkle with the garam masala and toss until evenly coated. Transfer to the prepared baking sheet, spread them into a single layer and season with salt and pepper to taste. Roast for 20 to 25 minutes, flipping the veggies halfway through.

Meanwhile, if using dried lentils, drain and rinse the lentils. Put them in a pot and add 1½ cups (355 ml) of water. Bring to a boil, then lower the heat and simmer until tender, 15 to 20 minutes. Drain and rinse under cold running water, then let them drain completely. (If you're using canned lentils, there is no need to cook them, but be sure to rinse and drain well.)

When ready to serve, arrange the arugula on a large platter (or divide between 2 plates or shallow bowls) and top with the lentils and roasted vegetables. Serve warm or at room temperature.

## serving suggestions:

- Top the salad with fresh herbs and seeds.

- Drizzle with lemon juice, Balsamic Vinaigrette (page 198) or Lemon-Tahini Sauce (page 199).

- Sprinkle with some Almond Ricotta (page 203).

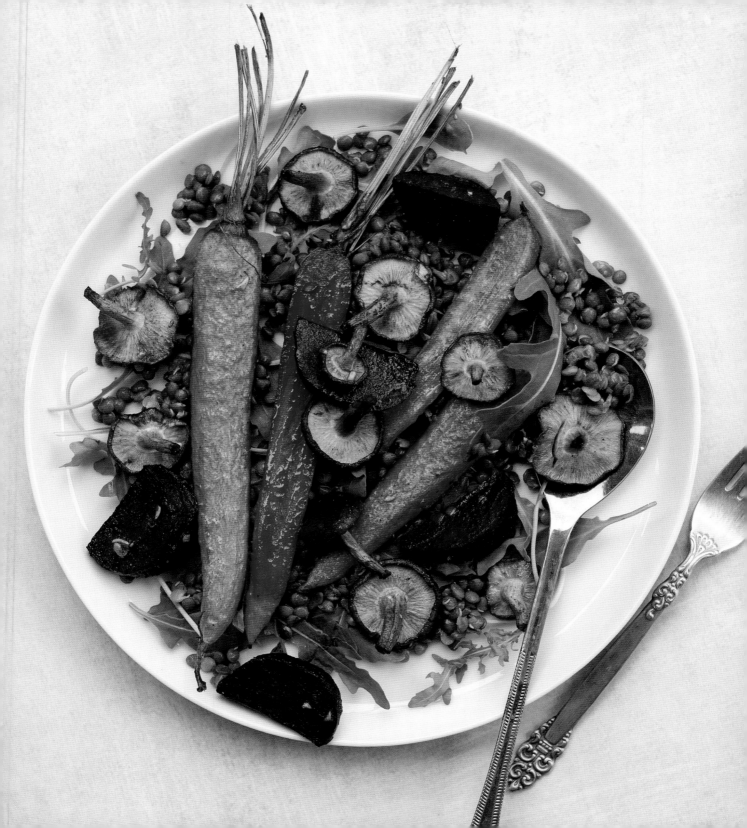

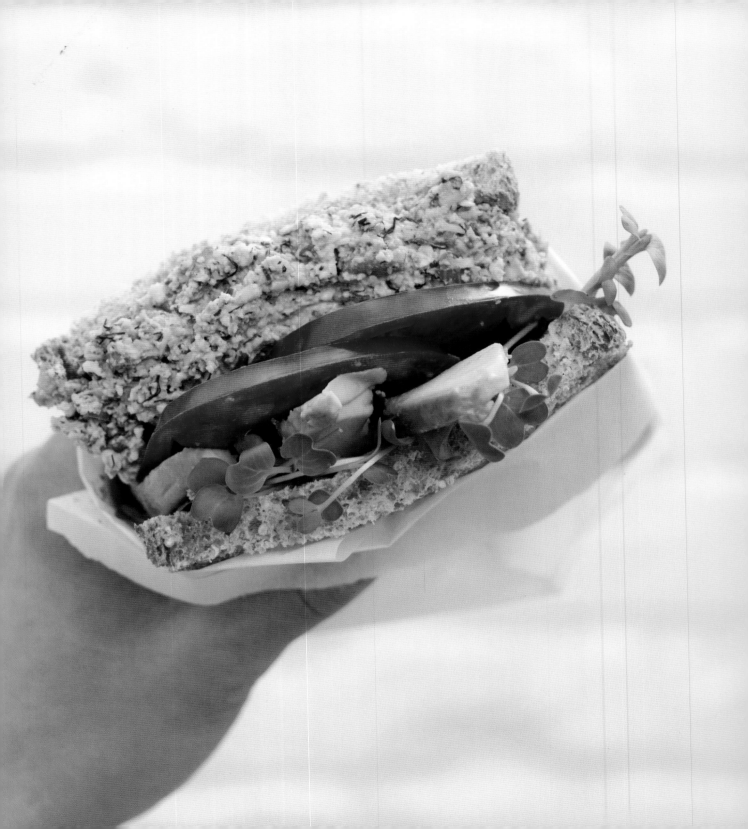

# mock tuna salad

Raw | mineral rich | thyroid support  •  Soaking time: 2 hours | Yields: 4 servings

A tuna salad without actual tuna may seem like a hard sell, and I have to admit that it took me a while to even experiment with this recipe, but once I got on board, it became one of my favorites! So, how can something taste like tuna when it is all raw and made from plants? The secret is dulse. Dulse provides the perfect mineral balance in a natural form and so is a superior source of minerals and trace elements we need daily for optimal health. Dulse is also rich in iodine, a key part of dietary health. Iodine helps with the formation of thyroid hormones, which regulate the body's energy production, promotes growth and development and helps burn excess fat. There are many other excellent health benefits, but let's stop right there so we can get busy in the kitchen!

## salad

2 cups (290 g) raw sunflower seeds, soaked in water for 2 hours (see notes)

3 to 4 ribs celery, diced

2 scallions, diced

2 tbsp (6 g) dulse flakes

¼ cup (15 g) fresh dill

## dressing

⅔ cup (117 g) hemp hearts

¼ cup (60 ml) coconut water or purified water

3 cloves garlic, peeled

½ cup (120 ml) fresh lemon juice

1 tsp sea salt

2 tbsp (30 ml) stone-ground mustard

Prepare the salad: In a food processor, puree the sunflower seeds until they are a slightly chunky pâté. Transfer to a bowl.

Mix in the celery, scallions, dulse flakes and dill. Stir well and set aside.

Prepare the dressing: In a blender, combine all the dressing ingredients and blend until smooth. Pour the dressing over the salad, toss to mix well and serve.

## serving suggestions:

Serve on sprouted-grain bread, on seedy crackers, in veggie wraps or on top of a basic leafy green salad. Or just enjoy it all on its own!

### notes:

- To soak the sunflower seeds, in a large glass or stainless-steel bowl, cover the seeds with 4 cups (946 ml) of water. Leave them on the counter to soak for 2 hours. After they are done soaking, drain and rinse them in a strainer.

- Look for dulse flakes in your local health food store. You could use kelp powder instead, if you can't find the dulse flakes.

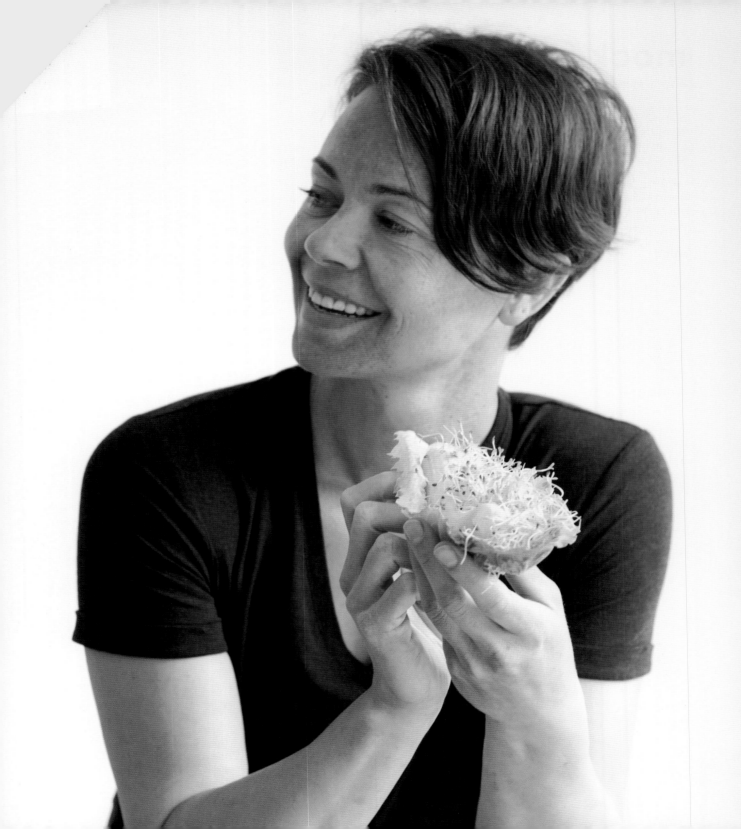

# one-minute
## meals

Even though we love our creative time in the kitchen, there are days we'd rather focus on other things than make a multiple-step meal with a bunch of ingredients. If you can relate, try one of these nine simple meal ideas. They are our simple go-to combinations that take less than five minutes to make, yet will help you feel energized, satisfied and nourished.

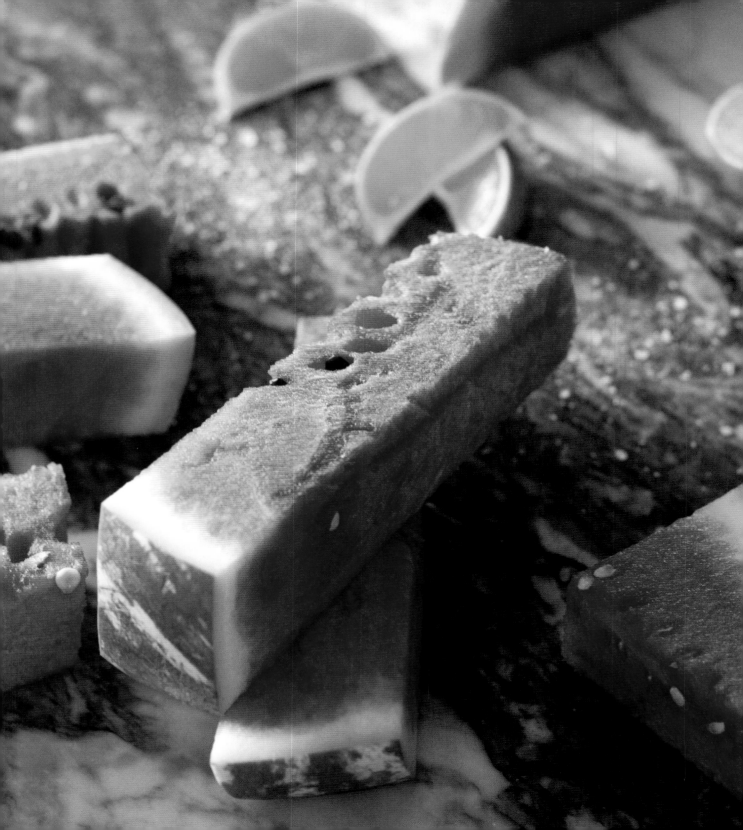

# watermelon + lime + sea salt

Yields: 2 servings

Watermelon's health benefits are beyond anything you could ever imagine—this fruit is a true healer! With a touch of fresh lime juice and a pinch of good-quality sea salt, you have yourself a perfect postworkout combination to help reduce muscle soreness and improve recovery.

¼ to ½ (8- to 10-lb [3.6- to 4.5-kg]) watermelon (depends on size of fruit)

½ lime

Pinch of Celtic sea salt

Cut the watermelon into sticks. Arrange on a plate, squeeze some lime juice onto it and sprinkle with sea salt.

# mango + hemp hearts

Yields: 1 serving

This meal is loaded with protein and healthy fat from the hemp hearts, plus provides fiber from the fresh, juicy mango. It's surprisingly filling and will help satisfy your sugar cravings any time of the day!

1 ripe mango, peeled, pitted and cut into chunks

1 tbsp (11 g) hemp hearts

Place the mango pieces in a bowl. Sprinkle with the hemp hearts and dig in!

> **note:**
> You can replace the mango with banana, blueberries or pineapple.

# pineapple + spirulina in a jar

Yields: 1 serving

Pineapple and spirulina is a match made in heaven! You get all the benefits of spirulina without that "spirulina taste." We love spirulina and do our best to include it in our daily diet. This natural algae powder is incredibly high in protein and a good source of antioxidants, B vitamins and other nutrients. When harvested correctly from uncontaminated ponds and bodies of water, it is one of the most potent nutrient sources available. Spirulina is primarily made up of protein and essential amino acids, and is a great natural way to boost your iron levels.

¼ pineapple, peeled and cut into bite-sized chunks

1 tsp organic spirulina powder

Fill a quart (1-L)-sized mason jar two-thirds full with the pineapple chunks. Add the spirulina powder. Close with a lid and give it a nice shake. Enjoy right away or keep in the fridge until ready to eat. This is also a convenient meal to pack with you for a busy day ahead.

# apple-tahini sandwich

Yields: 1 serving

A fun meal that can be quickly assembled by slicing an apple and topping it with a thin layer of raw tahini. Sprinkle with a tablespoon (11 g) of hemp hearts and a pinch of cinnamon, and you've got yourself a winner! These little sandwiches are high in protein, high in fiber and provide 40 percent of your daily iron needs.

1 medium apple (organic if possible)

2 tbsp (15 g) raw tahini

1 tbsp (11 g) hemp hearts

Ground cinnamon

Wash, core and slice the apple into 6 rounds. (If you don't have an apple corer, you can slice the apple first and then cut out the centers with a small cookie cutter or knife.)

Spread the tahini on 3 of the apple slices and sprinkle with the hemp hearts and a little bit of cinnamon. Top with the remaining apple slices to form sandwiches.

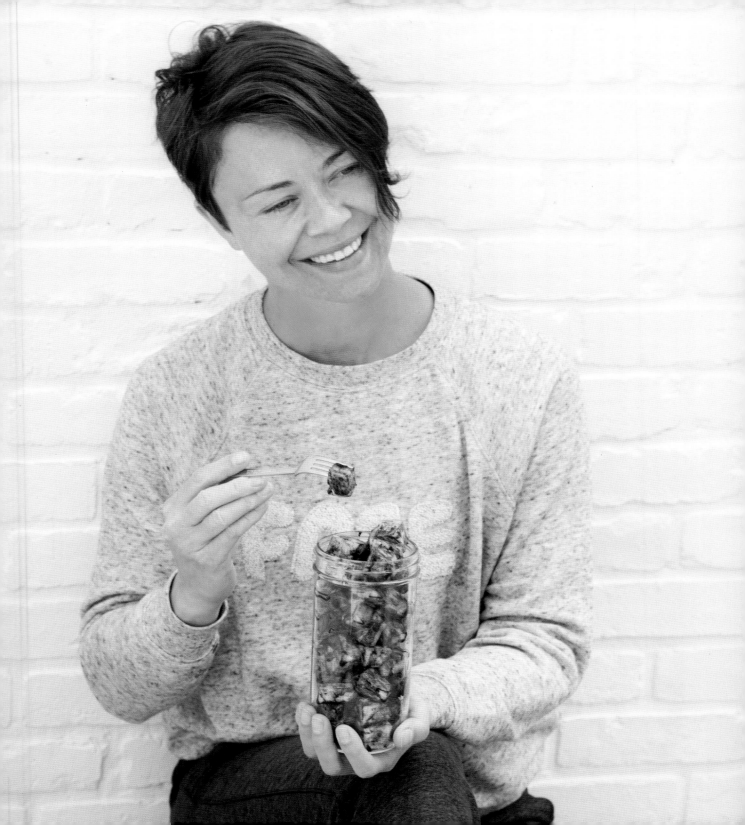

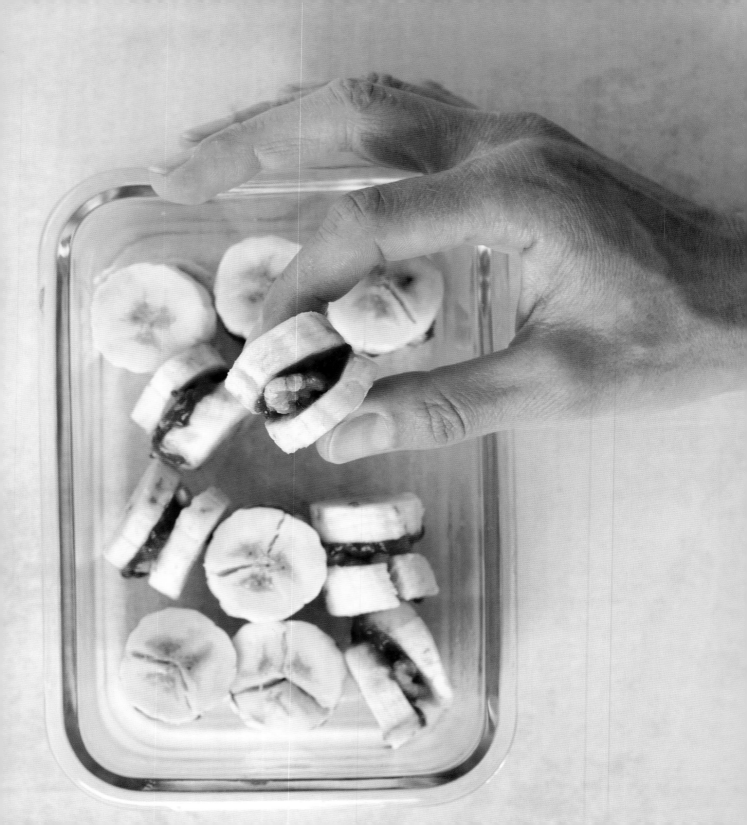

# jammed walnut banana bites

Yields: 1 serving

Candy bar cravings don't have to turn into a complete junk food bomb. Instead, slice a banana, chop some walnuts (or your nut of choice), add a touch of chia jam and you got yourself a quick snack that will satisfy your sweet tooth in a healthy and nourishing way.

1 banana

4 or 5 walnut halves

1 tbsp (15 ml) Simple Berry-Chia Jam (page 211)

Slice the banana into rounds (as you would for cereal—not too thin or else it may break). Put a walnut half on one piece of the banana and jam on another piece. Take the two banana rounds and create a little sandwich with them and devour!

# banana + nut butter + cacao nibs

Yields: 1 serving

This energizing snack is a healthy way to satisfy your sweet cravings and get in 10 grams of plant protein! We realize that banana and nut butter combo is nothing new, but somehow the addition of crunchy cocoa nibs makes them that much more satisfying. Great as a midday snack.

1 banana

1 tbsp (16 g) raw nut butter

1 tbsp (8 g) cacao nibs

Peel the banana and smear 1 side with the nut butter.

Sprinkle with the cacao nibs.

Slice and enjoy!

# dates + almond butter

Yields: 1 serving

Dates are a great fuel before, during and after training, providing high energy, iron and potassium. So, skip the premade snack bars and make this quick and healthy combo instead.

2 Medjool dates, pitted

1½ tsp (8 g) raw almond butter or other raw nut butter

Slice the pitted dates down the middle so just the bottom half is still attached (so you can open it).

Spread half of the almond butter between the 2 halves of each date and squeeze the dates back together. That's it!

# avocado + sprouts nori roll

Yields: 1 serving

Avocado toast is all the rage, but replacing the bread with a sheet of seaweed takes it to a new level! The addition of fresh alfalfa sprouts rolled inside this amazingly simple, yet nourishing meal is a great way to get your dose of BCAAs (branched-chain amino acids) and glutamine.

1 raw, organic nori sheet

½ avocado, peeled, pitted and sliced

Handful of alfalfa sprouts

Place the nori sheet, shiny side down, on a flat surface.

Down the center, add the avocado, then the sprouts.

Wrap the nori roll tightly, using a small amount of water to seal the last end together, then cut in half and eat immediately.


# banana + sprouts + romaine lettuce tacos

Yields: 1 serving

Yes, we admit that the combination of banana, sprouts and lettuce might seem a little odd, but we love it! It's fast, highly nutritious and delicious combo! Try it for yourself!

1 banana

1 large leaf romaine lettuce

Handful of sprouts

Place the banana inside the lettuce leaf and top it with any sprouts.

*See image on page 174.

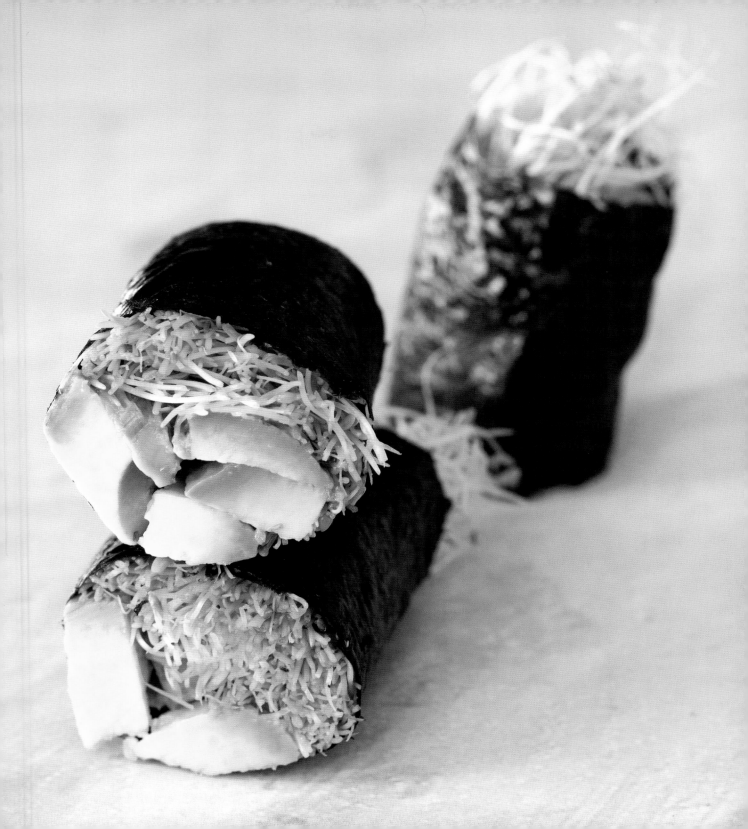

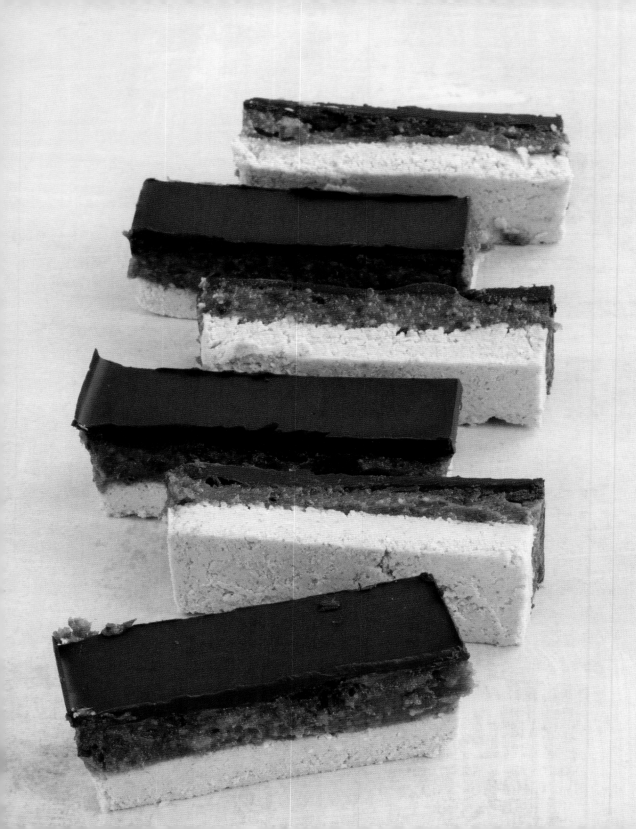

# desserts
## with benefits

It is possible for you to "have your cake and eat it too." We've compiled six dessert recipes that are packed with elite superfoods and intended to satisfy a sweet tooth, yet also deliver an easily digested energy-packed fuel source to help you move through your day unhindered by fatigue or indigestion. So, go ahead and indulge in a piece of Blackberry-Lemon Cheesecake (page 187) or a Nik's Twix Bars (page 188) and boost your body with health at the same time.

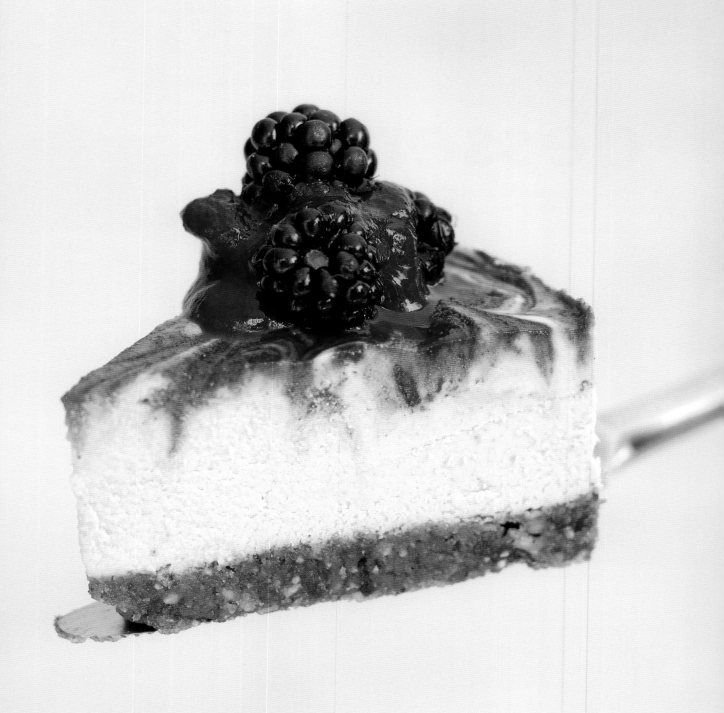

# blackberry-lemon cheesecake

Raw | promotes muscle recovery | high fiber • Soaking time: 4 hours (or overnight) | Yields: 1 (6-inch [15-cm]) round cake

This raw cheesecake uses only wholesome ingredients, and of course, like all our recipes, it's gluten- and dairy-free! Berries, figs, nuts and spices create this plant-powered treat that is rich in vitamins, minerals and enzymes present in the whole living foods. There is one particular ingredient that adds an extra nutritional punch, and that is lucuma. This low-glycemic sugar alternative delivers a subtle sweetness—along with vital health-boosting nutrients. If you have this superfood on hand, then mix it into the cheesecake to help boost your muscle growth as well as recovery.

## crust

1 cup (150 g) dried figs, diced

¾ cup (100 g) raw Brazil nuts

¼ tsp ground nutmeg

¼ tsp ground cinnamon

⅛ tsp Himalayan pink salt

## blackberry syrup

1 cup (145 g) fresh or frozen blackberries, thawed

5 Medjool dates, pitted

1 tbsp (15 ml) fresh lemon juice

## cheesecake filling

2 cups (280 g) raw cashews, soaked in water for at least 4 hours or preferably overnight

½ cup (120 ml) canned coconut milk, shaken

¼ cup (55 g) cacao butter or coconut oil, melted and cooled

⅓ cup (80 ml) raw agave nectar (see note)

½ cup (120 ml) fresh lemon juice

½ tsp vanilla bean powder, or 1 tbsp (15 ml) pure vanilla extract

1 tbsp (8 g) lucuma powder (optional)

## suggested topping

¼ cup (38 g) fresh blackberries, for decoration (optional)

Prepare the crust: In a food processor fitted with the S blade, process all the crust ingredients to a doughlike consistency—the final crust dough should hold together when you pinch it between your fingers.

Pat down the crust dough in an even layer on the bottom of a 6-inch (15-cm) round springform pan and set aside.

Prepare the blackberry syrup: In your blender, blend together all the syrup ingredients until smooth. Transfer the syrup to a small bowl and set aside.

Prepare the filling: Drain the soaked cashews and discard the water.

In a high-powered blender or a food processor, combine all the cheesecake filling ingredients and blend until creamy smooth. This process can take 2 to 4 minutes, depending on the strength of the machine.

Pour the batter into the pan over the crust. Gently tap the pan on the counter to remove any air bubbles.

Drop spoonfuls of the blackberry sauce all over the cheesecake (sort of in a checkerboard fashion) reserving some for serving if you wish.

To create the swirls, drag a wooden skewer or chopstick through the syrup puddles—this creates a beautiful, unique design.

Chill in the freezer for 4 to 6 hours; after that store in the fridge until ready to decorate with fresh blackberries around the edge.

You can store the cheesecake in the fridge for 3 to 5 days or up to 3 months in the freezer. Be sure that the container is well sealed to avoid any fridge odors.

### note:

Our choice of sweetener in this recipe is raw agave nectar, also known as agave syrup. You could replace the agave with an equal amount of pure maple syrup. Although technically not raw, maple syrup is a great source of manganese and zinc.

# nik's twix bars

Raw | stress relief | increases energy • Yields: 12 bars

It's candy bar time! Both of us grew up eating the classics—Mars, Skor, Reese's Peanut Butter Cups and Twix. Nowadays, we love re-creating our childhood favorites into treats you can feel good about putting into your body. Unlike the store-bought version, Nik's Twix Bars are made with just a handful of all-natural ingredients, but taste just as decadent. Even better, they're quick to prepare. We used maca powder in the caramel layer. Maca, a.k.a. Peruvian ginseng, is a turniplike root vegetable native to the Andean mountains. It is incredibly abundant in amino acids, phytonutrients, fatty acids, vitamins and minerals. Maca helps lower cortisol levels and can also improve sleep quality. See—even a candy bar can be healthy!

## base

1 cup (95 g) almond meal (or dried pulp from mylk, page 50)

1 cup (80 g) certified gluten-free rolled oats

½ cup (120 ml) Date Syrup (page 56)

2 tbsp (30 ml) melted coconut oil, plus more for pan

## caramel layer

20 Medjool dates, washed & pitted

¼ cup + 2 tbsp (67 g) hemp hearts

¼ cup (60 ml) purified water

2 tbsp (30 g) maca powder

¼ tsp Celtic sea salt

## chocolate layer

1 (80-g) vegan dark chocolate bar

Prepare the base: In a food processor, combine the almond meal, oats, date syrup and coconut oil. Blend until well mixed and the mixture sticks together. If needed, add more date syrup or coconut oil to achieve the right consistency.

Lightly oil a 9-inch (23-cm) square pan with coconut oil, pack the base firmly into the bottom of the pan and set aside.

Prepare the caramel layer: Using the same food processor, combine all the caramel ingredients and blend until a thick caramel-like texture forms.

Using a spatula, spread the caramel evenly on top of the base. Place in the freezer.

Prepare the chocolate layer: Using a double boiler, melt the chocolate. Once the chocolate is completely melted, remove the cake from the freezer. Evenly pour the chocolate over the caramel layer. Once it starts to solidify, you can score into 12 bars by lightly cutting through the chocolate. This will help you cut the bars all the way through once they are completely set and ready to serve. Keep in the fridge until ready to eat.

Store in a sealed container in the freezer for up to 1 month.

*See photo on page 184.

note:

To keep this recipe raw, use 80% (or higher) dark raw chocolate bars.

# seasonal fruit crumble

Source of omega-3s | high fiber • Yields: 6 to 8 servings

This fruit crumble is simple to prepare, nourishing enough to be eaten for a morning meal, easy to pack for a workday breakfast, yet still delicious to enjoy with a dollop of coconut yogurt for dessert. It's bursting with fresh, juicy fruit and includes flaxseeds, rich in omega-3s that deliver anti-inflammatory benefits. Feel free to make use of whichever seasonal fruit you love. We listed some of our favorite choices, but you can also mix and match all different kinds. For the sweetener, we used a bit of pure maple syrup, but it honestly doesn't need much at all because the fruit is so sweet on its own.

## crumble

1 cup (100 g) certified gluten-free oat flour (ground oats)

½ cup (40 g) certified gluten-free rolled oats

¼ cup (42 g) ground flaxseeds

½ tsp Himalayan pink salt

1 tsp ground cinnamon, plus more for coating (optional)

½ tsp ground cardamom

1½ tsp (3 g) grated fresh ginger

Zest and juice of ½ lemon

¼ cup (55 g) organic raw coconut oil

¼ cup (60 ml) pure maple syrup, plus more for coating (optional)

## filling

4 to 5 cups (750 to 850 g) fresh seasonal fruit, such as 5 large organic peaches, 3 organic pears + 2 cups (290 g) of mixed berries, or 5 large organic apples

Coconut oil, for pan

Preheat the oven to 350°F (180°C).

Prepare the crumble: In a large bowl, combine the oat flour, oats, ground flaxseeds, salt, cinnamon, cardamom, ginger, lemon zest and juice, coconut oil and maple syrup (if using) until fully combined with a crumblelike texture that sticks together. Set aside.

Prepare the filling: Wash, peel and slice the fruit, if necessary. Coat a 10-inch (25-cm) cast-iron baking pan or casserole dish with coconut oil.

If you wish, coat the fruit with cinnamon and a touch of maple syrup, depending on how tart or how sweet the fruit is and also your preference.

Spread the fruit evenly into the pan and cover with the crumble topping. Using a spatula or clean hands, gently press the topping down to compact it.

Bake for 40 to 50 minutes, or until lightly browned.

### note:

Serve as is or with Cultured Coconut Yogurt (page 55).

# golden banana bread

High fiber | anti-inflammatory  •  Yields: 10 servings

Are you craving a little home comfort? Satisfy your soul with this delicious and wholesome banana bread. It is moist, sweet and smells like heaven. We have made many healthy loaves of bread, and this combination of ingredients is simply amazing. The balance of flavors and texture is perfect, and the inclusion of turmeric gives it potent anti-inflammatory and cancer-fighting properties. An ideal reward after a hard training session!

Coconut oil, for pan

### dry ingredients

2 cups (190 g) almond meal (ground almonds)

1 cup (80 g) certified gluten-free rolled oats

¼ cup (42 g) ground flaxseeds

2 tbsp (10 g) whole psyllium husk

2 tsp (5 g) ground cinnamon

½ tsp ground turmeric

½ tsp Himalayan pink salt

### wet ingredients

4 very ripe bananas

¼ cup (60 ml) Date Syrup (page 56)

3 tbsp (45 ml) raw agave nectar

1 tsp vanilla bean powder

### suggested add-ins (optional)

½ cup (75 g) raisins

½ cup (50 g) chopped walnuts

1 cup (150 g) diced banana

### garnish (optional)

1 very ripe banana, sliced

¼ cup (44 g) chopped dark vegan chocolate

Preheat the oven to 375°F (190°C). Coat the bottom and sides of an 8½ x 4½-inch (21.5 x 11.5–cm) loaf pan with coconut oil.

Prepare the dry ingredients: In a high-speed blender or food processor, combine all the dry ingredients. Pulse together until well mixed, keeping some of the oats whole. Set aside.

Prepare the wet ingredients: Place the 4 bananas into a large bowl and, using a fork, mash until smooth. Add the date syrup, agave and vanilla bean powder and mix well. Next, add the dry mixture and mix until well combined. It should form a doughlike texture due to the ground flaxseeds and psyllium husk.

Mix in your choice of add-ins.

Scoop the dough mixture into the prepared pan and press firmly down to remove any air pockets. If you wish, slice a ripe banana into 4 pieces lengthwise and place side by side on top of the loaf.

Bake for 50 minutes. Check to be sure it is thoroughly done by poking it with a toothpick in the center. The toothpick should come out clean.

When done, remove from the oven and allow it to cool in the pan. Garnish with banana slices or chocolate, if using.

note:

Tastes great on its own or served with Power Nut Butter (page 58).

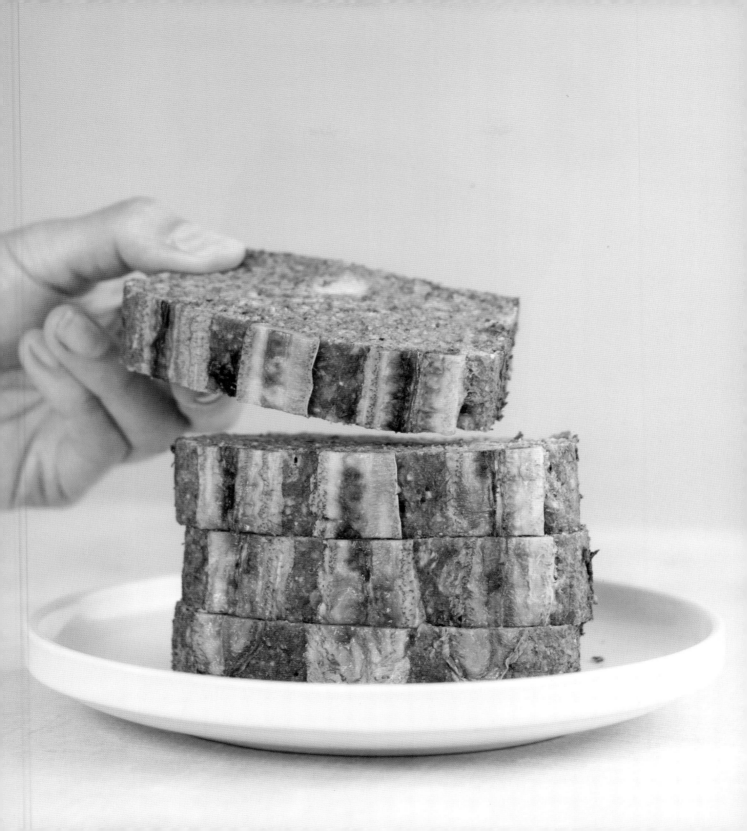

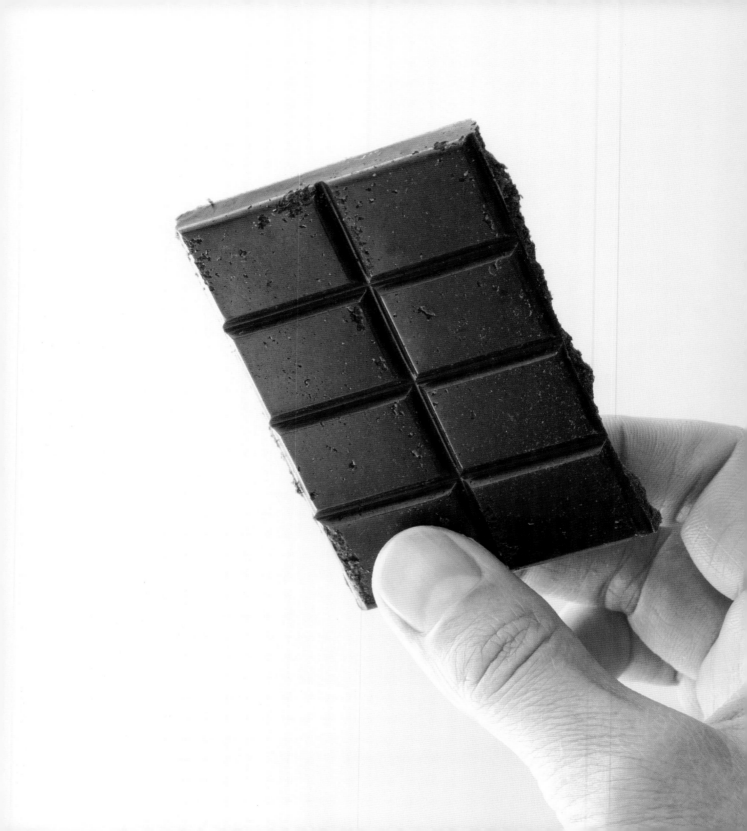

# ॐ om chocolate bar

Raw | high in antioxidants | mood enhancing • Yields: 1 chocolate bar

No matter how healthy and clean you eat, there might be some days when you want to inhale a nice bar of chocolate. So, why not! After all, chocolate has some amazing health benefits. However, hold on . . . before you rip open that Snickers bar loaded with junk (including processed sugar, soy lecithin, artificial flavor, corn syrup, milk fat, partially hydrogenated soybean oil, salt, egg whites and other food additives), consider creating a bar of healthy chocolate yourself. You see, the type of chocolate we benefit from is not the milk chocolate stuff many of us call chocolate. That's actually candy.

On the other hand, real chocolate—the high percentage of cocoa stuff—is one of nature's most potent antioxidant foods on the planet. It provides an abundant source of iron and magnesium, which support healthy heart function and may also improve cognitive performance. This raw chocolate bar is simple. It contains a triple threat of cacao (powder, butter and nibs), dates and sea salt—that's it. Understated, but once you try it, there's a good chance it'll become your new healthy addiction.

⅓ cup (59 g) Medjool dates, pitted (about 4 dates), or ⅓ cup (80 ml) Date Syrup (page 56)

3 tbsp (45 ml) purified water (if using whole dates)

1 cup (225 g) cacao butter

½ cup (55 g) cacao powder

2 tbsp (15 g) cacao nibs

Pinch of Celtic sea salt

## suggested toppings

Goji berries

Raisins

Hemp hearts

Macadamia nuts

Spirulina powder

Maca powder

If using whole dates, soak them in 1 cup (240 ml) of warm water for 10 minutes. Drain and place in a high-speed blender together with 3 tablespoons (45 ml) of purified water. Blend until a smooth, syruplike consistency is achieved. Set aside.

In a heat-safe medium bowl set over a saucepan partly filled with boiling water, gently melt the cacao butter over low heat. Remove from the heat, then add the cacao powder through a fine-mesh strainer to prevent clumping. Add the date syrup and stir to combine. Add the cacao nibs and salt and stir to incorporate evenly. Spoon into bar molds and sprinkle with your choice of toppings. Place in the freezer to harden. Remove from the molds and store in a covered container in the freezer or refrigerator.

Enjoy in moderation with good friends or family.

notes:

- Cacao production is labor and resource-intensive, and occurs in countries that may not protect workers or the environment. Commercial production can involve slave-type labor and deforestation. We encourage you to always buy organic and Fair Trade ingredients. Our go-to brand is Giddy Yo (see the resources section on page 216).

- I like to use silicone chocolate molds. They make it easy to remove the finished chocolates. They come in many different shapes and sizes. If you do not have chocolate molds, simply spread the chocolate mixture evenly on a parchment paper-lined pan.

# superfood caramels

Raw | iron rich | high in antioxidants  •  Yields: 12 pieces

These chewy chocolate-covered salted caramels come guilt-free. Tahini is ground sesame seeds—full of healthy fats and protein that nourish your body. Mixed with iron-rich dates to help combat anemia and a healthy dose of superfood powder, basically, this could be considered medicine. Right? Lucuma powder has a delicious maple flavor. It's high in fiber, B vitamins and beta-carotene (an antioxidant that helps combat free radicals) and potassium (great for workout recovery) and contains 14 essential trace elements, including high amounts of iron, calcium and phosphorous.

12 to 14 Medjool dates, pitted

½ cup (120 g) raw tahini

1 tbsp (8 g) lucuma powder

1 tsp Himalayan pink salt, plus more for sprinkling

1 (80-g) bar dark organic chocolate

In a food processor, combine the dates, tahini, lucuma and salt. Blend until well mixed; it should start to form a ball in the food processor.

Place the "caramel" on a piece of parchment paper and cover with another piece. Use a rolling pin to start to flatten it into a square or rectangular shape about ½ inch (1.3 cm) thick. Place in the freezer for at least 20 minutes, or until firm enough to cut.

Once the caramel is ready, please leave it in the freezer. Line a large plate with parchment paper and set near your stovetop.

In a double boiler or a heat-safe medium bowl set over a saucepan partly filled with boiling water, gently melt the chocolate over low heat, stirring occasionally to prevent the chocolate from overcooking. Once the chocolate is fully melted, lower the heat or turn it off. Next, remove the caramels from the freezer and place them on a cutting board. Cut into square or rectangular pieces that are the average size of a piece of caramel.

Using a spoon, carefully dip a caramel into the melted chocolate. Be sure to cover the whole piece. Place it on the parchment paper–lined plate.

Sprinkle the coated caramel with Himalayan pink salt before the chocolate hardens. Continue with the remaining pieces, then place the entire plate in the freezer.

Once the chocolate has hardened for at least 30 minutes, enjoy some pieces and place the rest into an airtight container and store in the freezer.

notes:

- The caramel inside the chocolates does not freeze completely, so you can eat them straight from the freezer.

- To keep this recipe raw, use an 80% (or higher) dark raw chocolate bar.

- Lucuma can be replaced with maca powder, baobab or mesquite.

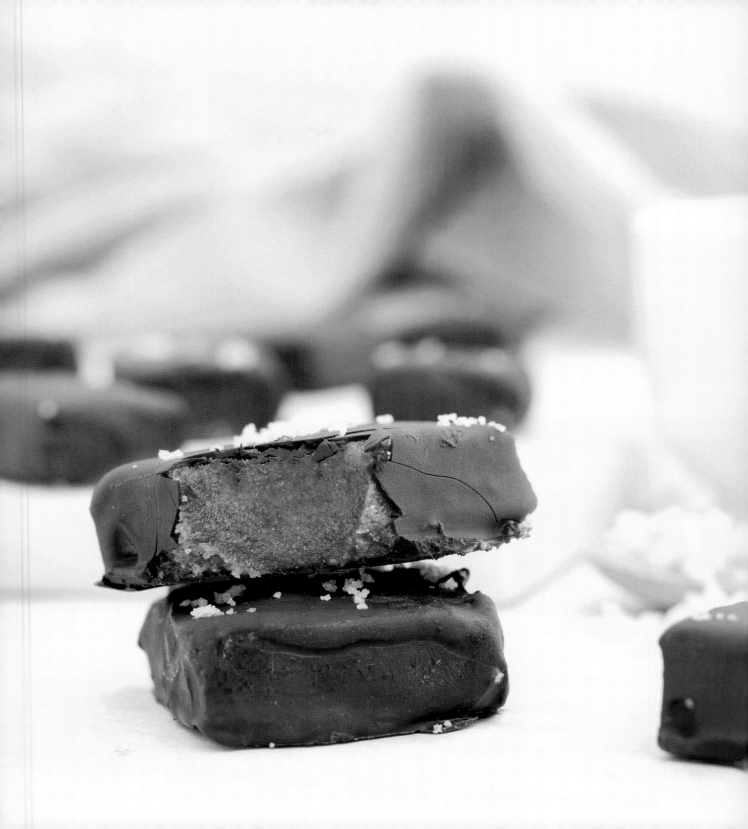

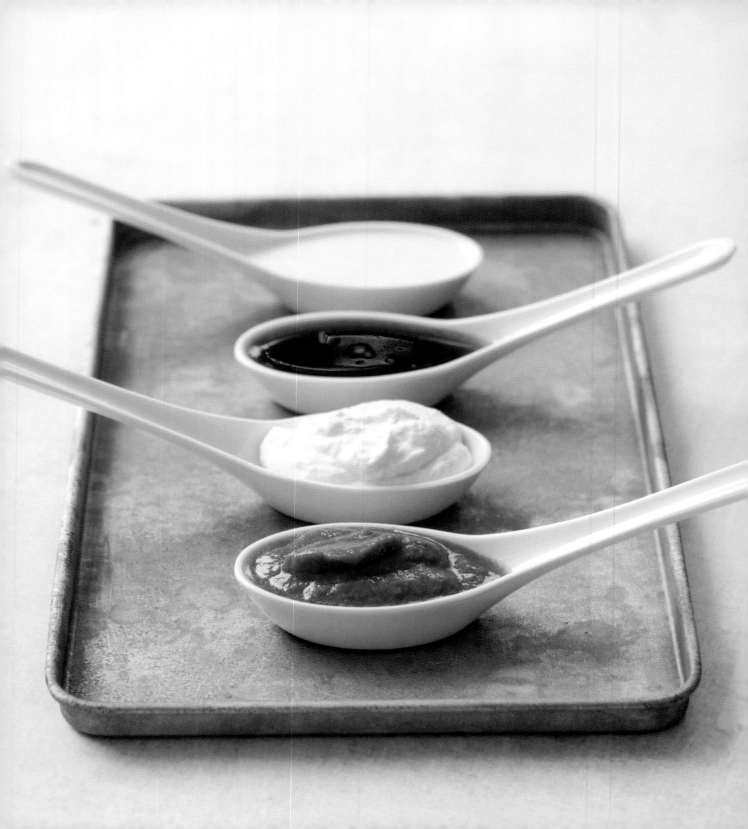

# dressings, dips, spreads and chutneys

A great sauce, dressing or dip can make all the difference between dull salad and rockin', mouthwatering meal. This lineup has some of the staple recipes that we've perfected over the years, and most of them can be made easily in several minutes! So, let's get ready to create some dairy-free sour cream (page 200), ricotta "cheese" (page 203), Cilantro Chutney (page 201), Three-Layer Party Dip (page 207), Lemon-Tahini Sauce (page 199) and so much more!

# balsamic vinaigrette

High in antioxidants | healthy joints   •   Yields: 1 cup (240 ml)

This basic balsamic vinaigrette is quick, easy, healthy and delicious! However, before we get to the recipe, let's talk balsamic vinegar for a second. Quality is key! Balsamic vinegar that comes in giant bargain bottles tends to be acidic and often contains caramel color and sweeteners. Instead, look for a smaller bottle of well-aged balsamic of Modena, meaning it has matured in wooden barrels for at least three years. How can you tell if it's a good-quality product? First, read the ingredients; it should not include caramel color or added sugars. Also, the bottle should have a yellow and blue IGP stamp, a certification guaranteeing it's made from grape varietals typical of Modena, Italy.

½ cup (120 ml) flax oil, hemp oil or extra virgin olive oil

½ cup (120 ml) high-quality balsamic vinegar

2 tbsp (30 ml) agave nectar

1½ tsp (8 ml) stone-ground mustard

Pinch of sea salt

In a lidded glass jar, combine all the ingredients in the order listed. Shake the jar vigorously until completely mixed.

Serve on your favorite salad or store in the refrigerator to use later; the dressing will keep for about 2 weeks. It might separate; just shake it up before using.

*See photo on page 196.

## serving suggestions:

- Of course, on salads.
- Drizzle over a quinoa dish.
- Drizzle over sweet potatoes and other roasted or raw vegetables.

# lemon-tahini sauce

Raw | easy to digest | iron rich  •  Yields: 1½ cups (355 ml)

This sauce is alkalizing, nutrition packed and dangerously addictive. The creamy texture of blended tahini with a few other basic ingredients creates a smooth, dairy-free yet rich sauce that can be spread, drizzled and added to pretty much anything.

1 cup (240 g) raw tahini

½ cup (120 ml) purified water, plus more, if needed

Juice of 2 lemons

1 tbsp (15 ml) cider vinegar

1 (1½" [4-cm]) piece fresh ginger, peeled

1 tsp ground coriander

1 tsp ground cumin

1 tsp fennel seeds

1 tsp salt

½ tsp freshly ground black pepper

In a blender or food processor, combine all the ingredients (starting with only ½ cup [120 ml] of water) and blend until smooth. Gradually add some more water, blend again and continue until the dressing reaches your desired consistency.

The dressing will keep for 4 to 5 days in the fridge.

*See photo on page 196.

## serving suggestions:

- Drizzle over chopped up raw greens and salads.
- Use as a dip for fresh or roasted vegetables.
- Serve as a sauce for falafel and veggie burgers.
- Use as a spread for sandwiches and wraps.

## pro tips:

- You can make this sauce into a salad dressing by simply adding a couple extra tablespoons (15 ml or more) of purified water.
- Make sure to use a raw tahini that has no other ingredients added.

# clean sour cream

Raw | muscle food | bone health  •  Soaking time: 2+ hours | Yields: 1 cup (240 g)

How can you make a dairy-free and healthy "sour cream"? The answer is soaked nuts. Especially macadamias and cashews! Once soaked, these two nuts blend into a smooth and creamy texture that closely resembles cream cheese. I have tried making this sour cream with both kinds of nuts, and my personal preference is the macadamia version. I quite enjoy the unique flavor of macadamias, plus these delicious nuts are considered a muscle-building food! One cup (135 g) contains 11 grams of protein and all the essential amino acids, which are critical for overall health and muscle growth. Okay, enough about nuts—let's get to this simple and yummy recipe . . .

1 cup (135 g) macadamia nuts or (140 g) cashews, soaked in water for 2+ hours or overnight

½ cup (120 ml) purified water

2 tbsp (30 ml) fresh lemon juice

¼ cup (60 ml) cider vinegar

1 tsp onion flakes

½ tsp sea salt

Drain and rinse the nuts well.

In a high-speed blender, combine all the ingredients and blend until smooth.

Store in an airtight container in the fridge for 4 to 5 days.

*See photo on page 196.

**note:**

If you do not have a high-powered blender, such as Vitamix, make sure you soak the nuts for 8 to 12 hours to achieve a smooth, creamy texture. The longer you soak, the more water they'll absorb and less extra liquids will be needed in the actual recipe. Less water will result in thicker sour cream, whereas more water will make it thinner. Keep in mind that refrigerating will also thicken your sour cream.

## serving suggestions:

This sour cream goes great on everything:

- Sprouted Falafel (page 153)
- Walnut Meat Lettuce Tacos (page 144)
- Smoky Tempeh Scramble (page 91)
- Warming Tortilla Soup (page 136)
- Salads
- Sandwiches

# cilantro chutney

Raw | anti-inflammatory | digestive aid  •  Yields: ¾ cup (204 g)

This chutney, made with fresh ingredients, is a simple yet flavorful sauce that can be enjoyed with many different dishes. Two bonuses: It only takes a few minutes to prepare and it will last in the fridge for a few days. The star of this recipe is cilantro. This herb is one of the top sources of chlorophyll that promotes alkalinity in the body and aids with digestion, hormone balance and ridding the body of excess mercury and lead. Another powerful ingredient that gives this chutney a mildly spicy flavor is ginger. We include ginger into our diet pretty much daily as it promotes healthy digestion; it's an effective anti-inflammatory and antioxidant that helps prevent muscle pains and osteoarthritis.

1 big bunch cilantro

½ cup (75 g) green raisins

⅓ cup (78 g) cubed fresh pineapple

1 (½" [1.3-cm]) piece fresh ginger, grated

¼ tsp ground cumin

2 tsp (10 ml) cider vinegar

Pinch of freshly ground black pepper

½ tsp Celtic sea salt

Clean the cilantro under running water and remove any thick stalks (for this recipe, we only want leaves and extremely thin stalks).

In a small food processor or blender, combine all the ingredients. Blend well to create a smooth fine chutney.

Transfer to a bowl or glass jar and serve.

Keep leftovers in an airtight container in the fridge for 3 to 4 days.

*See photo on page 196.

## serving suggestions:

This chutney can be enjoyed with a variety of dishes, such as:

- Sprouted Falafel (page 153)
- Walnut Meat Lettuce Tacos (page 144)
- As a dip with crackers
- On top of zoodles (zucchini noodles)
- Drizzled over salads and bowls

## pro tip:

When buying fresh herbs, such as cilantro, choose a bunch that has a vibrant green color and that holds straight when held upright. If it droops, it's not fresh and will affect the taste of the chutney.

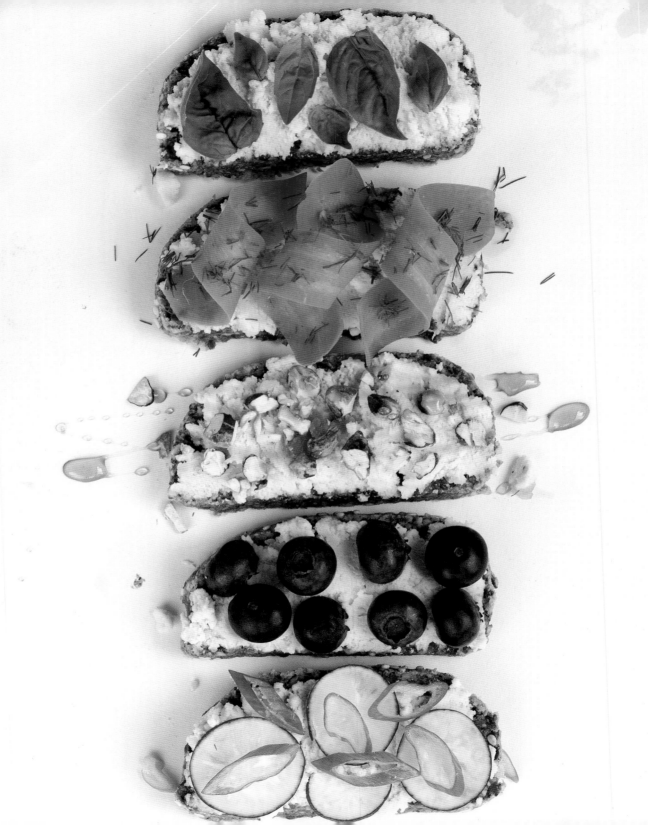

# almond ricotta

Fermented | immunity boosting | digestive aid   •   Soaking time: 2+ hours |
Yields: 2 cups (500 g)

This almond ricotta provides loads of nutrition and makes a unique and versatile addition to your plant-powered meals. Growing up in Europe, I believe I have developed a bit of a cheese addiction. This ricotta is creamy and slightly sweet in flavor, just like traditional ricotta! Although it takes a little bit of time to make, it's worth the extra effort.

2 cups (290 g) almonds, soaked in water for 2+ hours

1½ cups (355 ml) purified water

1 tsp Celtic sea salt

1 to 2 probiotic capsules

Drain and peel the soaked almonds (see notes).

In a high-speed blender, combine the purified water and salt, then add the almonds. Blend until smooth and creamy.

Pour the mixture though a cheesecloth or nut milk bag and allow to drain for 4 hours or overnight.

Transfer the drained mixture to a clean glass bowl or container. Break open the probiotic capsule(s) and using a wooden or plastic spoon gently stir it in.

Cover with a clean towel and leave to ferment for 8 to 12 hours at room temperature. Use this timing as a basic range. The culturing process can go slower or quicker than expected, depending on the environment. Taste the cheese throughout the fermenting process to find the optimal flavor that you prefer. Be sure to use a clean spoon each time so you don't contaminate the cheese.

Once fermentation is complete, you can add other ingredients, such as lemon juice, garlic, freshly ground black pepper, herbs, sun-dried tomatoes or even dried fruit.

Store in the fridge in an airtight container for up to 2 weeks. The longer the cheese ages in the fridge, the tangier it will taste.

notes:

- Removing the skin gives the almonds a smooth texture, which is helpful in making such dishes as this one. To begin, soak your almonds for 2 hours or overnight, drain and rinse well. Use your fingers to gently squeeze the almonds and loosen the skin from them. Once all almonds are peeled, rinse them again and now they are blanched and ready to use in your recipe.

- The number of capsules you use will depend on the strength of the probiotic. The probiotic that we currently use for fermentation is Natren Megadophilus Dairy Free Capsules, available at most natural food stores. However, you can use any brand that you have on hand.

# mango salsa

Raw | promotes healthy gut | helps prevent anemia  •  Yields: 4 servings

A blend of the three primary tastes: sweet, sour and spicy, this raw salsa is as simple as just mixing the ingredients. No blending, no cooking. Originally, I created this recipe to pair with the Sprouted Falafel (page 153), which worked out to be an excellent match. However, this salsa could easily be enjoyed as a side salad or added to your Nourish Bowl (page 146).

2 raw mangoes (preferably very ripe)

½ cup (90 g) diced tomato

½ cup (70 g) diced cucumber

¼ cup (40 g) finely chopped onion

Juice of 1 lime

1 tsp fennel seeds

1 tbsp (10 g) chia seeds

Handful of fresh mint leaves, finely chopped

⅛ to ¼ tsp cayenne pepper, or more to taste

¼ tsp Himalayan pink salt

Peel the mangoes. Place a mango on its side, with the stem facing you, so that it's standing on its narrow side, not the broad side. Insert your knife just to the right of center and cut off the side, tracing the contour of the pit with your knife. Repeat with the other half.

Trim off the remaining mango around the pit, then cut the mango into ¼-inch (6-mm) cubes. Repeat with the second mango.

In a bowl, combine all the ingredients and gently toss, making sure everything gets well coated with the flavorings. Adjust the spices according to taste and serve.

Store leftovers in the fridge for 2 to 3 days.

## serving suggestions:

- Perfect as an appetizer with raw veggies

- Goes nicely with Sprouted Falafel (page 153)

- On top of a salad or Nourish Bowls (page 146)

- Inside lettuce wraps and tacos (page 144)

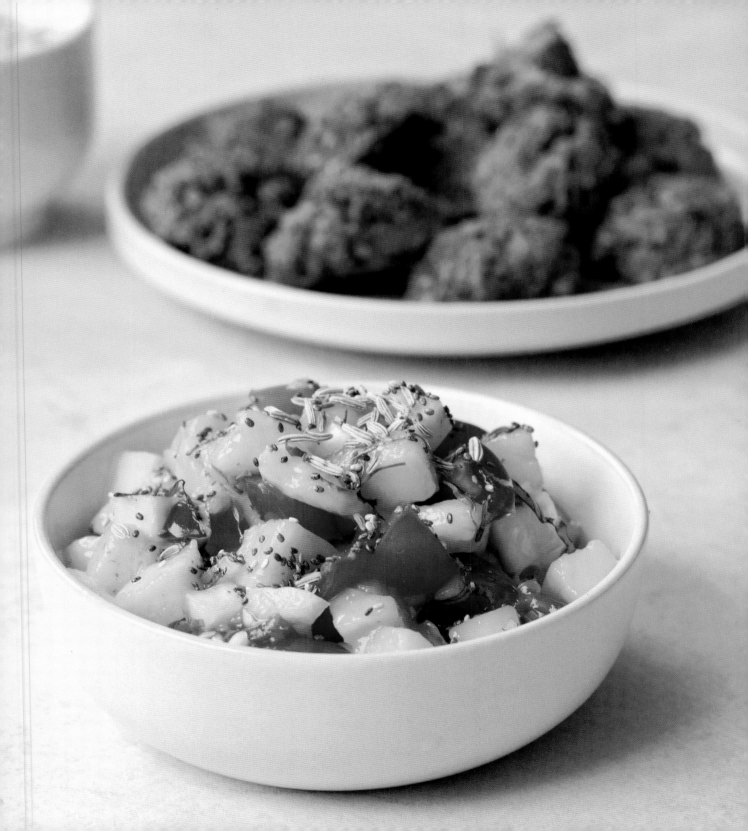

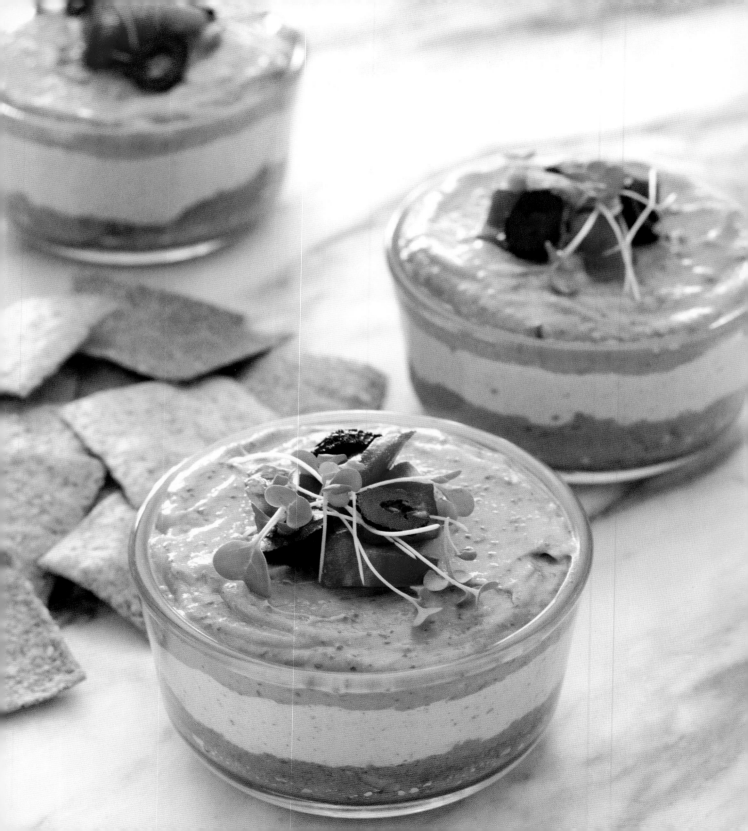

# three-layer party dip

*Raw | protein rich | bone health* • Soaking time: 2+ hours | Yields: 5 or 6 servings

With traditional dips, you end up eating empty calories that are hard on the digestive system and the waistline. The next time you host a party or have company over, serve this upgraded version of layered dip instead. The whole dish is made entirely from scratch, but don't let that discourage you. The process is pretty simple and mostly involves mixing things in a food processor. We like to use small individual serving-sized bowls. However, you could prepare this in a large glass dish as well.

## "refried beans"

1 cup (145 g) sunflower seeds, soaked in water for 2 hours

¼ cup (14 g) sun-dried tomatoes, soaked in water for 30+ minutes

½ cup (120 ml) purified water, or more if needed

1 tsp ground cumin

1 tsp sea salt

1 tbsp (3 g) dulse flakes

1 tsp smoked paprika

## "cheese sauce"

1 cup (140 g) raw cashews, soaked in water for 2 hours

¼ cup (60 ml) fresh lemon juice

1 large yellow bell pepper, seeded and roughly chopped

½ cup (64 g) nutritional yeast

¼ tsp cayenne pepper

2 cloves garlic

1 tsp turmeric

1 tsp Himalayan pink salt

1 tbsp (7 g) ground flaxseeds

## guacamole

2 avocados, halved, pitted and peeled

Juice of 2 limes

½ tsp Himalayan pink salt

¼ tsp freshly ground black pepper

¼ cup (10 g) fresh cilantro, roughly chopped

## suggested toppings

Chopped tomatoes

Sprouts

Sliced black olives

Chopped green onions

Prepare the "refried beans": After soaking the sunflower seeds and sun-dried tomatoes, drain them and place in a food processor fitted with the S blade. Process until they start to break down.

Add the water, cumin, salt, dulse flakes and smoked paprika and process until almost smooth but with a little texture, much like refried beans. Distribute the mixture evenly into the bottom of the bowl(s) of your choice.

Prepare the "cheese sauce": Be sure to soak the cashews for at least 2 hours; this will help soften the nuts to make a smooth, creamy sauce. Drain and rinse when ready to use.

In a high-powered blender, combine all "cheese sauce" ingredients and blend until creamy. Spread the mixture smoothly over the "refried beans."

Prepare the guacamole: In a food processor, combine all the guacamole ingredients and blend until smooth. Spread on top of the dip.

Garnish with any additional toppings of your choice.

Serve immediately or cover and refrigerate. Can be made up to 1 day in advance.

## serving suggestions:

This goes great with:

- Fresh-cut veggies
- Crisp endive leaves (just gently rinse and pat dry before serving)
- Sprouted-grain chips or crackers

# roasted beet dip

Mineral rich | digestive support | helps lower swelling  •  Soaking time: 8 hours |
Yields: 2 cups (480 g)

This dip is supersimple, superdelicious and much easier to digest than traditional hummus. It's all the things we love a dip to be—creamy, packed with flavor and good for you! Beets nourish the blood and tonify the heart, can help protect against cancer, are good for anemia and relieve constipation. On top of that, they are a perfect pre- and postworkout fuel. Our favorite way to enjoy this party-friendly recipe is by dipping into it with fresh-cut veggies or spreading it inside nori wraps. It pairs well with our Simple Nut & Seed Bread (page 63) too.

2 medium or 3 small red beets

½ cup (73 g) sunflower seeds, soaked in water for 8 hours

1 tbsp (15 ml) hemp oil

Juice of 1 lemon

2 tbsp (30 ml) balsamic vinegar

1 tsp fennel seeds

½ tsp sea salt

½ tsp freshly ground black pepper

Preheat the oven to 400°F (200°C). Wrap the beets in unbleached parchment paper and place them on a baking sheet. Roast for 30 to 40 minutes, or until the beets are fork-tender.

When cool enough to handle, peel away the beet skins, using your hands. Chop the beets and place them in a blender or food processor. Add the remaining ingredients and blend until smooth.

Store in an airtight container in the fridge for up to 5 days. Leftovers make the perfect weekday lunch solution or take-along snacks.

## serving suggestions:

- As a dip for raw veggies and any nut & seed crackers
- Great as a spread for the Veggie Nori Rolls (page 143) or sandwiches

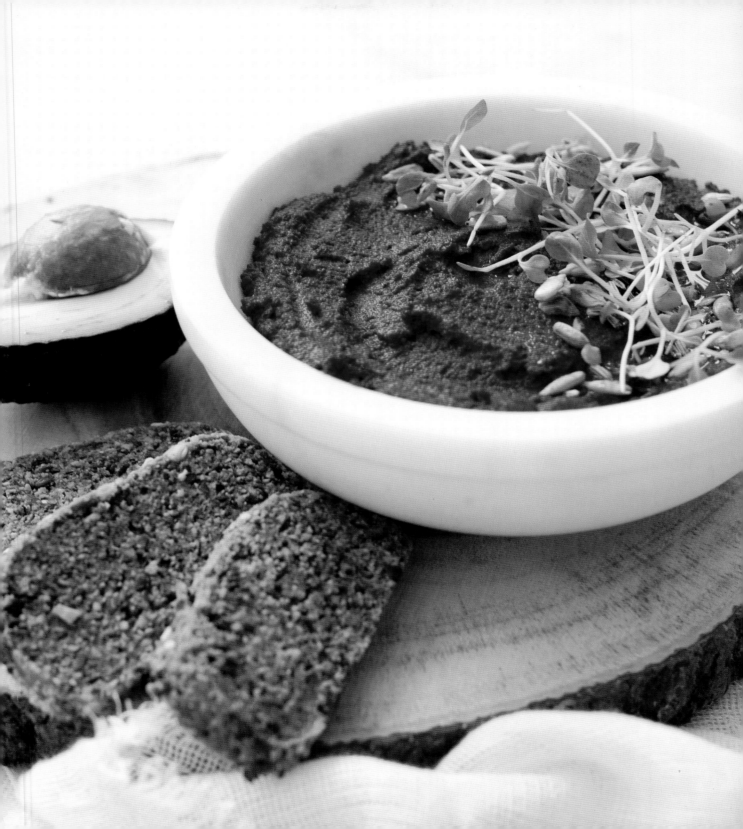

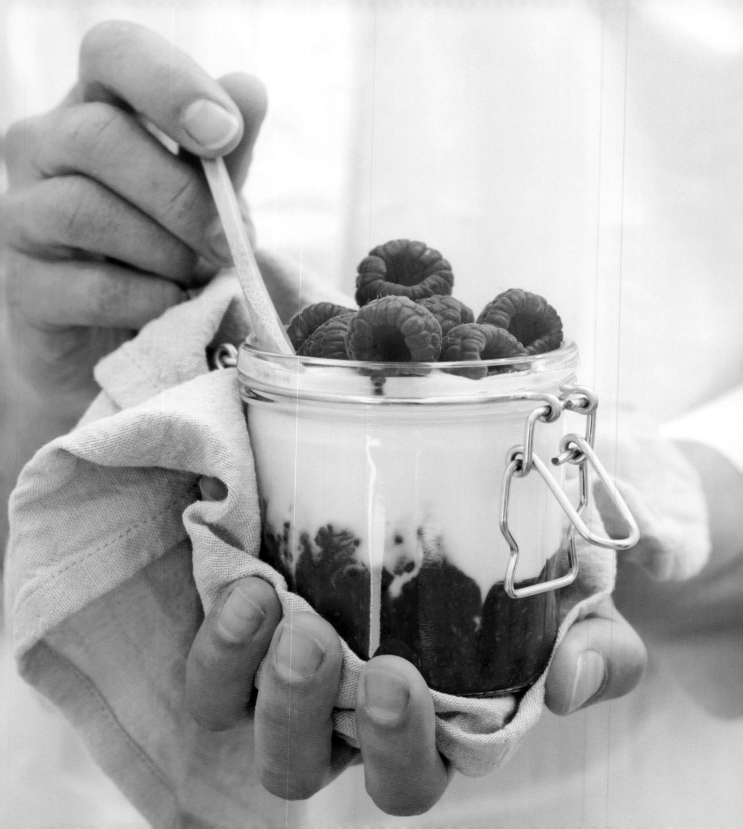

# simple berry-chia jam

Raw | high in antioxidants | energy boost    •    Yields: 1½ cups (432 g)

Berries are one of the best foods on Earth, containing significant amounts of antioxidants, vitamin C, manganese and fiber. Unfortunately, most of these incredible nutrients are lost when the fruit is exposed to high heat during processing. This simple raw jam maintains all the heat-sensitive antioxidants and enzymes, and it's a great alternative to an overprocessed and sugar-loaded store-bought variety.

2 cups (290 g) frozen organic berries, any variety or a mixture

1 tsp fresh lemon juice

2 tbsp (20 g) chia seeds

1 to 2 tbsp (15 to 30 ml) Date Syrup (page 56) or agave nectar (optional)

In a food processor, pulse the berries until well chopped but not pureed.

Add the lemon juice, chia seeds and syrup (if using) and pulse just to combine.

Place in an airtight jar or container and refrigerate overnight; the jam will thicken.

That's it! Store in the fridge for 5 to 7 days.

## serving suggestions:

- Spread on sprouted-grain toast.
- Mix it with coconut yogurt.
- Drizzle over a smoothie bowl.

## notes:

- Raw jams are best made in small batches. Extra jam that can't be finished in 5 to 7 days can be stored in the freezer.

- You can replace the berries with other fruits; just adjust the amount of chia seeds used, which will depend on how juicy the fruits are.

- Aim for organic berries if you can, as nonorganic berries are high on the list for absorbing pesticides. Organic fruit also tends to be higher in nutrients than conventionally grown fruit.

# sample menus

## PLANT-POWERED ENDURANCE MEAL PLAN

**UPON WAKING** - 24 oz (720 ml) pure water (or Cleansing Morning Lemonade [page 71])

**PRE-WORKOUT** - Cucumber-Lime Chia Fresca (page 96) or Creamy Mango-Chia Pudding (page 87)

**DURING WORKOUT** - Salted Caramel Endurance Gel (page 118)

*(workouts longer than 60 minutes)*

**POST-WORKOUT** - Postrun Juice (page 100)

**SNACK** - 1 cup (240 ml) Cultured Coconut Yogurt (page 55) and 2 tablespoons (11 g) goji berries

**LUNCH** - Pesto Quinoa Bowl (page 150)

**SNACK** - 2–3 pieces of organic fruit

**DINNER** - Roasted Vegetable & Lentil Salad (page 170)

**DESSERT** - 1–2 Raw Cinnamon Rolls (page 129)

**SNACK** - Sleep Tonic (page 115)

# PLANT-POWERED
# MUSCLE BUILDING MEAL PLAN

**UPON WAKING** - 24 oz (720 ml) pure water (or Cleansing Morning Lemonade [page 71])

**PRE-WORKOUT** - Banana or Dates + Almond Butter (page 181)

**POST-WORKOUT** - Blood Transfusion Juice (page 103) or Pineapple + Spirulina in a Jar (page 178)

**SNACK** - Raw Power Smoothie (page 104)

**LUNCH** - "The Game Changer" Burger (page 157) with Green Mix Salad (page 59)

**SNACK** - 2-3 pieces of organic fruit

**DINNER** - Wild Rice Salad (page 169)

**DESSERT** - 2-3 Superfood Caramels (page 194)

**SNACK** - ½ English cucumber and apple

# PLANT-POWERED
# BEGINNER MEAL PLAN

**UPON WAKING** - 24 oz (720 ml) pure water (or Cleansing Morning Lemonade [page 71])

**BREAKFAST** - Avocado & Pea Smash (page 90)

**SNACK** - Morning Energizer Smoothie (page 79)

**LUNCH** - Greek Salad in a Jar (page 166)

**SNACK** - Epic Power Orbs (page 126)

**DINNER** - Nourish Bowl (page 146)

**DESSERT** - Apple-Tahini Sandwich (page 178)

# recovery tips and tools

During my career as a fitness coach, I have worked with many people who go full blast all the time, juggling a full-time job and family while taking sports seriously and working ambitiously to achieve their athletic goals. I get it. If we want to better ourselves physically and mentally, hard training is essential, long sessions are sometimes important and moving the body every day is a necessity. However, if our day-to-day life becomes all about performance and not about enjoying the ride, we're at risk of burning out and losing all joy and quality in what we're doing.

## Love yourselves enough to take time to rest and rejuvenate.

Rest and self-care are essential to finding balance in life. It serves as an armor to protect the energy that you need to survive and thrive. Attending to your body's needs is not selfish. On the contrary; listening to your body and creating balance goes a long way in managing stress, avoiding injuries and living your best life.

## Sunshine

A healthy dose of sunlight is medicine. To enjoy good health, build muscle and strength or even lose weight, it's essential to get adequate sunshine. Unfortunately, we have been conditioned to believe that the sun is dangerous and that the damaging effects of sunlight on the skin far outweigh any benefits. Public health campaigns reinforce this message in an attempt to reduce the annual increase in skin cancers. At the same time, it's estimated that over 70 percent of North Americans are deficient in vitamin D—a macronutrient that our body makes from cholesterol under the skin when exposed to the sun. This deficiency is one of the root causes of many diseases, including osteoporosis, heart disease, diabetes and cancer. When combined, the number of people who die from these conditions is far greater than the number of deaths from skin cancer, which is why the current take on sunlight needs, in my opinion, to be reevaluated. Recent studies are also finding that the standard American diet and exposure to the sun under the influence of alcohol or other diuretics, such as coffee, tea and soft drinks, dramatically increases the chances of damaging the skin. Personally, I chose to eat a clean plant-powered diet and make sure to get outside and honor the sun every single day.

### Sun exposure:
- Improves muscle development
- Promotes eye health
- Better bone health
- Increases metabolism/weight loss
- Improves sleep
- Enhances the immune system
- Reduces the risk of certain cancers
- Relieves stress

## Dry Brushing

Quickly brush your whole body with a dry body brush made of natural bristles or a good natural loofah. Start from your feet, brushing your skin upward toward the heart. This brushing method improves circulation, strengthens and rejuvenates the skin and helps with lymph drainage.

### Dry brushing:
- Increases muscle tone
- Improves skin texture (luminosity and suppleness)
- Supports natural detoxification
- Improves lymphatic circulation
- Enhances blood circulation
- Stimulates areas that accumulate cellulite

## Epsom Salts Baths

Have an Epsom salts bath after a hard training session to help with muscle soreness and recovery. Even one Epsom salts bath a week can have an incredible impact on your health.

- Magnesium helps relax skeletal muscles, aids in the absorption of vitamins and helps regulate muscle and nerve function.
- Add 1 cup (250 g) of Epsom salts to your next postworkout soak. Allow the body to relax for 30 minutes. Use this time to reflect on and appreciate all the positive aspects of your life.

## Cold Showers/Ice Baths

Yea, it's going to suck, but freezing your butt off for a few minutes is worth the initial discomfort. The general idea behind the ice-cold therapy is that exposure to cold helps to speed up the recovery process, after intense periods of physical activity by reducing inflammation and lactic acid buildup, while increasing blood flow and circulation of nutrients.

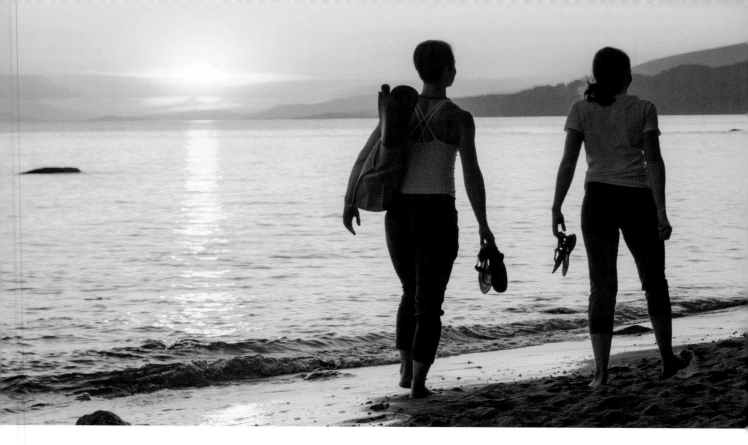

- Cold therapy reduces delayed onset muscle soreness.
- It also improves emotional resilience—cold showers and ice baths train your nervous system to be more resilient to stress.
- For an ice bath, add 1 bag of ice to your cold water bath postworkout. Build up time by 5-minute increment—not recommended longer than 20 minutes.

## Inversions

If you practice yoga, you have likely heard of this term. Inversions include all things that literally have you turning things upside down, from shoulder stand or headstand to legs up a wall. These are all inversions, and you do not need to be a superyogi to incorporate them into your daily life. Simply lying down with your legs up a wall will have you reaping the benefits of inversions. You can also take it to a different level and use a supportive sling to invert. We use something similar and find it incredibly beneficial.

### Inversion:
- Improves circulation of the blood and lymph
- Provides gentle passive stretching
- Reduces tension in the spine
- Increases joint mobility and flexibility
- Energizes
- Promotes good health and well-being

The human body is the most incredible system in the world and the ultimate feedback mechanism. The key to creating balance in every aspect of your life can be found by listening to your body and finding time to rest. Too much work can be as bad as not enough work. If your body is asking for something, you must follow its advice.

# helpful resources

## Online Support

The end of this book is the beginning of your plant-powered journey. To help encourage you on your path, we have created the following resources:

- Seasonal Produce Guide (free download)
- The Plant-Based Solution: 24-Week Guided Program
- Strong & Lean: Six Week Workout + Nutrition Plan
- 21 Days of Guided Meditation
- Fermentation for Beginners Course
- How to Sprout and Grow Microgreens: The Beginner's Guide
- 3-Day Juice Cleanse

All of these resources, as well as additional recipes and other helpful tools, are available for you at www.activevegetarian.com. Enter code PLANT-POWERED and receive 25 percent off all online programs.

## Recommended Books

Here are some of my favorite books for gaining a deeper understanding of the science and research behind the whole food, plant-based diet and its many benefits.

### The Natural Way to Vibrant Health
### by Norman W. Walker

Dr. Walker is a pioneer in plant-based diets and one of my health heroes. He lived to be 99 years old and wrote several books that have had a profound effect on my life. If you have not read any of his books, I encourage you to start reading them.

### Timeless Secrets of Health and Rejuvenation
### by Andreas Moritz

I'm extremely grateful for Andreas Moritz and the work he did to provide us with knowledge on how to improve overall health and well-being. He wrote several amazing books, and this one, in particular, has enhanced my life in so many ways. It's packed with over 500+ pages of information about the human body and the underlying causes of disease. If you are ready to dive deep into health and well-being, you will enjoy this book.

### The Thrive Diet
### by Brendan Brazier

Brendan Brazier is a leader in the modern plant-based nutrition for athletic performance. As a former endurance athlete, he offers great insight into how you can be strong and perform at your best while eating plant-based. The recipes in this book are created with the purpose to help energize, fuel and support recovery. A great guide for your health, and your kitchen.

## Recommended Documentaries

These two documentaries are showcasing the power of a plant-based diet on athletic performance. Very inspiring!

### The Game Changers

A fantastic documentary with a Hollywood-style budget, produced by James Cameron. It does a great job of demonstrating how a plant-based diet is changing the game in sports, health and other areas. It's engaging, informative and entertaining the whole way through. We highly recommend it to any athlete or nonathlete who cares about his or her health.

### From the Ground Up

This documentary goes quite in depth and follows the story of a former meat-eating college football player Santino Panico as he prepares for a marathon on a vegan diet. It explores how vegans recover quicker, have less inflammation, can work out more often and compete at the top levels of athleticism, including the MMA, NFL, professional running, surfing, skateboarding and triathlons.

## Our Favorite Food Companies & Products

This is a list of companies that make high-quality products that will help you create the *Plant-Powered Athlete*'s recipes.

### Giddy Yo

Giddy Yo is not your typical company. Not only does it hand craft delicious vegan, organic raw dark chocolate, it also offers spirulina, chlorella, goji berries, clean coffee, cacao, local medicinal mushrooms and other superfoods. As a reader, you are eligible for a 20 percent discount off regular-priced goods and free shipping for orders that are $75 or more. Use code ACTIVEVEG (www.shop.giddyyoyo.com).

## Upaya Naturals

This online superstore offers a large selection of high-quality organic superfoods, nuts, seeds, spices and grains as well as vitamins and kitchen equipment. It's definitely worth checking out. You can use the code ACTIVEVEG and receive $20 off your first order of $100 or more (www.upayanaturals.com).

## Harmonic Arts

An excellent selection of top-quality wild-harvested herbs, a variety of seaweed, medicinal mushrooms, loose teas and more! We have been using this company's products for many years, and love the quality and variety it offers. The owners are very knowledgeable and inspiring, and their customer service is top-notch. If you purchase directly from their website and use the code ACTIVEVEGETARIAN, you will receive 20 percent off your order (www.harmonicarts.ca).

## Kitchen Equipment to Get You Started

This list includes the appliances we have in our kitchen; however, you do not need them all to get started on the Plant-Powered Diet.

## Vitamix Blender

A high-quality blender is one of the essential kitchen tools that will help you succeed with your plant-powered journey. We use a Vitamix machine and can honestly say that for the past fifteen years, it has been the most versatile and most reliable kitchen appliance we have owned. Many of the recipes in this book, including soups, sauces, smoothies and energy gels, require the use of a blender. Vitamix has the horsepower to muster through leafy greens, dense dried superfoods, frozen fruits and whole nuts and seeds without leaving chunks and pieces unprocessed. The manufacturer offers a wide range of performance levels from personal blending to commercial use, so you can find the one that suits your needs. Available online at www.vitamix.com.

## Omega J8006 Juicer

We juice almost every day and often start the morning with a big glass of fresh juice and some days have another one after our training session. Over the last ten years, we have tested probably dozens of different juicers, and this Omega juicer is our top pick. If you are not ready to invest in a juicer, you can get away with using your Vitamix blender to do the job. Just blend the juice ingredients with a cup (240 ml) of water and then strain through a nut milk bag. However, if you want a high-quality fresh juice, the Omega J8006 is a great choice. Available online at www.omegajuicers.com.

## Cuisinart 14-Cup Food Processor

This versatile machine is convenient for making nut butter, dips, walnut meat and bread. Cuisinart also offers smaller models. However, I find that a 14-cup (3.3-L) version is a good size for processing things like cabbage or vegetables used to make sauerkraut and salads.

## Excalibur Food Dehydrator

A dehydrator is certainly not essential for your plant-powered lifestyle; however, for anyone interested in experimenting with raw living foods, this kitchen appliance works wonders. A dehydrator is essentially a low-temperature oven that slowly draws moisture out of food without cooking it. And when I say slowly, I mean it. The recipes in this book that have the option to use a dehydrator require between 4 and 8 hours of dehydrating, so be sure to make a note of this before beginning a recipe.

# acknowledgments

We want to acknowledge the many leading experts, pioneers and healers whose work and writings on the subject of plant-based nutrition and vibrant living paved the path for this book—Dr. Norman Walker, Andreas Mortiz, Arnold Ehret, Dr. Robert Morse, Dan McDonald and Brendan Brazier, to name only a few. Without them, this book could not have been written—or at least would not have contained as vast a discussion on nutritional health.

We give sincere gratitude to Marissa Giambelluca, Meg Palmer and the entire team at Page Street Publishing for their dedicated effort, valuable advice and beautiful design of this book.

Jenna Jones, our lifestyle photographer: Thank you for your keen eyes and chill attitude. Your photographs are gorgeous.

Finally, we must thank you, the reader, for investing your time and money into this book. We hope you enjoy it, and we hope you discover at least one thing that will leave a positive imprint on your precious life.

# about the authors

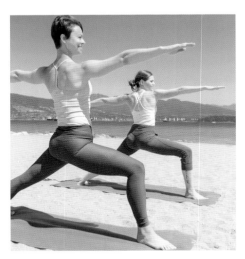

Zuzana Fajkusova and Nikki Lefler are health coaches, founders of ActiveVegetarian.com and authors of *Vegan Weight Loss Manifesto*; podcast hosts of their show, The Active Vegetarian; and celebrity trainers, yoga teachers and plant-based chefs. Zuzana & Nikki together have been plant-based for more than 20 years. Their deep passion for this lifestyle has led them to help others realize their health and fitness goals. They live a minimal life by the beach in Vancouver, Canada.

Instagram - @activevegetarian
Facebook - @activevegetarian
Pinterest - @activevegetarian

# index